Principles and Practice of
INTRAVENOUS THERAPY

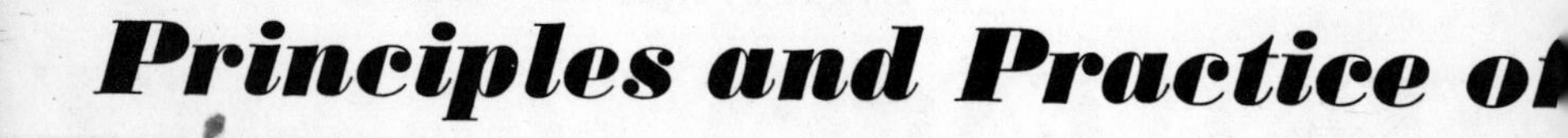
Principles and Practice of

NTRAVENOUS THERAPY

Ada Lawrence Plumer, R.N.

Supervisor and Instructor, Intravenous Department,
Massachusetts General Hospital, Boston

LITTLE, BROWN AND COMPANY, BOSTON

Library of Congress catalog card No. 74-127125

ISBN-0-316-71131(P)
ISBN-0-316-71130(C)

First Edition

Sixth Printing

Printed in the United States of America

Preface

THIS BOOK WAS WRITTEN in response to the need that became evident from giving instruction to nurses in intravenous therapy. The lack of information on this important therapeutic procedure was emphasized by the large number of intravenous nurses who attended the seminar "Incompatibilities of Parenteral Solutions," sponsored by the University of Connecticut recently.

In the past intravenous therapy consisted chiefly of supplying necessary fluid to the fasting patient. Today it is much more complex and involved. Its use is extensive, and it is now an integral part of the daily treatment of medical and surgical patients. Frequently it is a lifesaving procedure; safe and successful therapy is essential. This demands special knowledge and skill. Yet in spite of the increasing use and importance of parenteral therapy, little training is required of the average therapist to carry it out. It is considered sufficient by some that the therapist be able to perform a venipuncture. This does not contribute to the optimal care of the patient whose prognosis depends upon intravenous therapy. The purpose of this book is to present a source of practical information essential to safe and successful therapy.

Our knowledge of fluid and electrolyte balance has increased; we now recognize an imbalance as a threat to life—

a potential danger to the patient. This understanding has brought about an increase in the use of intravenous therapy and thus in the responsibility of the nurse. Knowledge of the fundamental concepts governing fluid and electrolyte balance contributes to safe therapy; knowledge of the endocrine response to stress assists the nurse to a better understanding of imbalances and problems associated with them. The nurse becomes alert to potential fluid and electrolyte disturbances, how they develop, and symptoms by which they are recognized.

Advances in drug therapy have further complicated intravenous therapy. The venous route offers pronounced benefits but is accompanied by problems and complications not existing in other forms of drug therapy. Very often the responsibility of compounding intravenous additives is left entirely to the nurse. With the continuous increase in drug products and parenteral fluids, the number of possible drug combinations is astronomical. This increases the likelihood of potential incompatibilities. Some basic knowledge should be available to those who share this responsibility.

Blood administration is an integral part of intravenous therapy. Rapid advancement in transfusion therapy increases responsibility for administering this vital fluid. The therapist shares responsibility for safe administration. She must know the disadvantages as well as the advantages associated with blood and its components; she must be trained in the proper handling of blood and the basic principles of its safe administration. Knowledge of the fundamental principles of immunohematology provides a basis for understanding the problems associated with blood administration. It alerts the nurse to potential reactions, why they develop, and symptoms by which they are identified.

No matter what type of therapy is involved, an understanding of the basic principles of safe fluid administration is vital. With any infusion there is a certain element of risk. The therapist and the nurse involved in fluid maintenance must know the potential hazards and how to prevent their occurrence.

The patient's prognosis may depend upon his ability to

receive a prolonged course of therapy. Preservation of the veins is important. Intravenous therapy may be given almost indefinitely if the therapist is skillful in (1) the choice of veins, (2) technique, and (3) the selection of proper equipment. The efficiency of the therapist may prevent the need of venous cut-downs and preclude the risk of adding the complication of thrombophlebitis to present illness.

With the increase in intravenous therapy, there is a definite need for parenteral teams. More and more hospitals are establishing intravenous departments. In addition to the technique and training essential to their function, this book also provides information on the organization of a team of intravenous nurses and the various duties that can be performed by this specialized group.

A. L. P.

Boston

Acknowledgments

I WISH TO EXPRESS MY DEEP APPRECIATION to Grant V. Rodkey for reading the entire manuscript and offering valuable comments and suggestions, and to all those other individuals listed for their cooperation, help, and interest in reading and critiquing specific chapters or sections of chapters:

GRANT V. RODKEY, M.D., Associate Visiting Surgeon, Massachusetts General Hospital

DONALD P. TODD, M.D., Anesthetist, Massachusetts General Hospital
Technique of Intravenous Therapy
Venous Pressure

BENJAMIN A. BARNES, M.D., Assistant Surgeon, Massachusetts General Hospital
Fundamental Aspects of Fluid and Electrolyte Metabolism
Rationale of Fluid and Electrolyte Therapy

JOHN F. BURKE, M.D., Visiting Surgeon, Massachusetts General Hospital; Chief of Shriners Burn Institute
Parenteral Therapy for the Burned Patient

JOHN W. WEBB, Director of Pharmacy and Supplies, Massachusetts General Hospital
Intravenous Administration of Drugs

SUE BRITTEN, B.Sc., First Research Technician, Blood Bank, Massachusetts General Hospital
Basic Immunohematology

MORTEN GROVE-RASMUSSEN, M.D., Director of Blood Bank and Transfusion Service, Massachusetts General Hospital
Transfusion Therapy

CHARLES HUGGINS, M.D., Associate Director of Blood Bank and Transfusion Service, Massachusetts General Hospital
Transfusion Therapy

SIDNEY V. RIEDER, Ph.D., Chief of Clinical Chemistry Laboratories, Massachusetts General Hospital
Laboratory Tests

MARY RUSSELL, Head Technician, Blood Bank, Massachusetts General Hospital
Blood Types

My appreciation is extended to the authors and publishers who have kindly allowed me the use of copyrighted material.

I am grateful to the Massachusetts General Hospital for giving me the opportunity to pioneer a program of intravenous therapy, one that has grown in thirty years from one nurse, myself, to the present thirty intravenous therapists.

Special thanks go to the intravenous nurses Jane Shea, Myra Ayer, and Stephanie Hayutin for their patience, helpful suggestions, and assistance in the development of this book.

A. L. P.

Contents

Principles and Practice of
INTRAVENOUS THERAPY

1.
Introduction

HISTORY OF INTRAVENOUS THERAPY

The idea of injecting various substances, including blood, into the circulatory system is not new; it has been in the mind of man for centuries. In 1628 William Harvey's discovery of the circulation of the blood stimulated increased experimentation. In 1656 Sir Christopher Wren, with a quill and bladder, injected opium intravenously into dogs, and six years later, J. D. Major made the first successful injection in man [4].

In 1665, an animal near death from loss of blood was restored by infusion of blood from another animal. In 1667 a 15-year-old Parisian boy was the first human being to receive a transfusion successfully; lamb's blood was administered directly into the circulation by Jean Baptiste Denis, physician to Louis XIV [4]. The enthusiasm aroused by this success led to promiscuous transfusions of blood from animals to man with fatal results, and in 1687 animal-to-man transfusions were prohibited.

About 150 years passed before serious attempts were again made to inject blood into man. James Blundell, an English obstetrician, revived the idea. In 1834, saving the lives of many women threatened by hemorrhage during childbirth, he proved that animal blood was unfit to inject into man and that only human blood was safe. Nevertheless complications persisted;

infections developed in donor and recipient. With the discovery of the principles of antisepsis by Pasteur and Lister, another obstacle was overcome, yet reactions and deaths continued.

In 1900, Karl Landsteiner, proved that not all human blood is alike; classifications were made [4]. In 1914 a chemical, sodium citrate, was found to prevent blood from clotting [4]. From then on rapid advance has taken place.

Administration of parenteral fluids by the intravenous route has become widely used only during the past thirty years. The difficulty in accepting this procedure was due to lack of safe solutions. The solutions used contained substances called pyrogens, proteins which are foreign to the body and not destroyed by sterilization. These caused chills and fever when injected into the circulation. About 1923, with the discovery and elimination of these pyrogens, the administration of parenteral fluids intravenously became safer and more frequent.

Until 1925 the most frequently used parenteral solution was normal saline solution. Water, because of its hypotonicity, could not be administered intravenously and had to be made isotonic; sodium chloride achieved this purpose [1]. After 1925 dextrose was used extensively to make isotonic solutions and to provide a source of calories [1].

In the early 1930's administration of an intravenous injection was a major procedure reserved for the critically ill patient. The doctor performed the venipuncture assisted by a nurse. The success of intravenous therapy and the great increase in its use led to the establishment of a department of specially trained personnel for infusion therapy. In 1940 the Massachusetts General Hospital became one of the first hospitals to assign a nurse as Intravenous Therapist. The services of the intravenous nurse consisted solely in administering intravenous solutions and transfusions, cleaning infusion sets, and cleaning and sharpening needles.

As our knowledge of electrolyte and fluid therapy grew, more solutions became available. Normal saline was no longer the only electrolyte solution, and today solutions are available to meet every need of the patient. Improvements and innovations in equipment have reduced hazards; sets and needles are now disposable, reducing risks of pyrogenic reactions and hepatitis.

With the increasing numbers of new drugs for administration by the venous route, and the increasing use of blood and its components, has come a corresponding need for infusion and transfusion therapy. Intravenous therapy now plays a vital role in the daily treatment of medical and surgical patients.

We have come a long way since 1940 when one nurse answered 3300 calls a year. The department at the Massachusetts General Hospital now consists of thirty highly skilled nurses who answer approximately 4000 calls weekly. The services performed by them are many:

1. Administration of parenteral fluids
2. Preparation and administration of drugs in solution
3. Administration of blood and its components
4. Performance of phlebotomies under supervision of the physician
5. Administration of hypodermoclysis
6. Collection of venous blood samples for all laboratories, e.g., chemistry, bacteriology, hematology, blood bank
7. Insertion of Levin tubes
8. Computation of blood volumes by means of the Volemetron

The administration of intravenous solutions may eventually become a requirement in the training of every registered nurse.

LEGAL STATUS OF INTRAVENOUS ADMINISTRATION BY NURSES

More and more of the responsibility for administering parenteral fluids is being allocated to the nurse. These responsibilities are not uniform but vary among hospitals and states. With the rapid advances in intravenous therapy, many large hospitals have recognized the need for skilled personnel and have organized parenteral teams; smaller hospitals in which resident physicians are not available are training their senior student nurses to perform venipunctures for injections of parenteral fluids.

Because this special function had been performed by the physician it was not previously considered a nursing procedure. Because it carries with it a certain element of risk and requires skill and knowledge to reduce the risk, many states have made formal rulings concerning its performance.

In 1961 an American Nurses' Association survey of rulings on the administration of intravenous procedures by registered nurses, showed that rulings had been made by state boards of nursing in six states and by attorneys-general in fifteen; other states indicated that the matter was determined by hospital policy or common practice. In some states the nurse practice acts relating to the definition of nursing are broad in wording and do not refer to specific procedures, because it is felt that since practice changes rapidly it would be unfortunate if certain procedures had to be reviewed by state legislators before appropriate personnel could carry them out.

Some states have joint policy statements on a number of procedures, including intravenous therapy (see Table 1). This

TABLE 1. States Having Issued Joint Policy Statements as of 1966

State	Name of Statement	Participating Groups
Arizona	I.V. Administration of Fluids Including Blood by Professional Registered Nurses (1962)	Arizona State Nurses Association Arizona Medical Association Arizona Hospital Association
California	Intravenous Administration of Fluids, Including the Starting and Administration of Blood by Registered Nurses (1957, amended 1965)	California Nurses Association California League for Nursing California Medical Association California Hospital Association

TABLE 1—*Continued*

State	Name of Statement	Participating Groups
Colorado	Intra-Cath Intravenous (1964)	Colorado Nurses' Association Colorado Medical Society
	Intravenous Medications (1965)	Colorado Nurses' Association Colorado Medical Society Colorado Hospital Association
Maine	Venipuncture Procedure by Licensed Professional Nurses (1964)	Maine State Nurses Association Maine League for Nursing Maine Medical Association Maine Hospital Association
Maryland	I.V. Administration of Fluids, Blood, Medication by Professional Registered Nurses (1965)	Maryland State Nurses Association Maryland Medical Society
Massachusetts	Administration of Intravenous Fluids by Professional Registered Nurses (1965)	Massachusetts Nurses Association Massachusetts League for Nursing Massachusetts Heart Association Massachusetts Medical Society Massachusetts Hospital Association Massachusetts Board of Registration in Nursing
Michigan	Venipuncture and Intravenous Administration of a Foreign Substance (1965)	Michigan Nurses Association Michigan State Medical Society

TABLE 1—*Continued*

State	Name of Statement	Participating Groups
New Mexico	Intravenous Administration of Fluids (Including Blood) by Professional Registered Nurses (1964)	New Mexico Nurses Association New Mexico Hospital Association New Mexico Medical Society
New York	Insertion of Intravenous Catheters (1966)	Medical Society of the State of New York Hospital Association of New York State
North Dakota	Joint Statement on the Intravenous Administration of Fluids and Medications by Licensed Professional Nurses Practicing in North Dakota (1965)	North Dakota State Nurses Association North Dakota Medical Association North Dakota Hospital Association
Ohio	Intravenous Therapy (1962)	Ohio State Nurses Association Ohio State Board of Nursing Education and Nurse Registration Ohio Department of Health Ohio Department of Mental Hygiene and Correction Ohio Hospital Association Ohio League for Nursing Ohio State Medical Association Ohio State Medical Board
Oregon	The Role of the Professional Nurse in Parenteral Therapy (1963)	Oregon Nurses Association Oregon Association of Hospitals Oregon Medical Association

TABLE 1—*Continued*

State	Name of Statement	Participating Groups
Pennsylvania	A Statement of Policy on the Intravenous Administration of Fluids (1960)	Pennsylvania Nurses Association Pennsylvania League for Nursing Pennsylvania Medical Society Pennsylvania Osteopathic Association Hospital Association of Pennsylvania
Vermont	Statement of Agreement on Venipuncture Procedure for Licensed Professional Nurses (1965)	Vermont State Board of Nursing Vermont Board of Medical Registration Vermont Medical Society Vermont State Nurses Association Vermont Hospital Association
West Virginia	I.V. Therapy Statement (1963)	West Virginia Nurses Association West Virginia League for Nursing State Board of Examiners for Registered Nurses State Board of Examiners for Practical Nurses West Virginia State Hospital Association West Virginia State Medical Association West Virginia State Society of Osteopathic Medicine Medical Licensing Board

type of statement is the result of deliberations by practitioners of nursing and medicine who are official representatives of the state nurses' association and state medical society. This is con-

TABLE 2. Massachusetts Joint Policy Statement

The Massachusetts Nurses Association and the Massachusetts League for Nursing in 1965 issued a Joint Statement Concerning Administration of Intravenous Fluids by Professional Registered Nurses. The following joint statement is set forth with the objective of providing for the health and welfare of the patient, and protecting the doctor, the nurse and the employing agency. The Massachusetts Nurses Association and the Massachusetts League for Nursing believe that it is a proper part of the practice of professional registered nurses to start and administer prescribed fluids intravenously (by needle) provided that:

1. The professional registered nurse, licensed to practice nursing in Massachusetts, should have had special, competent teaching in the technique;
2. Performance of the technique should be upon the order of a licensed doctor of medicine;
3. The order should be written for a specific patient;
4. Where the technique is to be performed in a hospital or any organized agency, the procedure should be performed within the framework of designated preparation and practice of the nurse established for the hospital or agency by a committee composed of representatives from the medical staff, the department of nursing and the administration; this framework of preparation and practice to be reproduced in writing and made available to every member of the medical and nursing staffs; and
5. It should be within the jurisdiction of that committee in a hospital or organized agency to:
   a. Decide if the nurses in the hospital or agency may perform the technique;
   b. Establish inservice teaching of the technique;
   c. Delineate the types of fluids that nurses may administer;
   d. Keep an approved list of medications that may be added to the fluid by the nurse and provide an inservice program that will acquaint the nurse with the reactions, contraindications, dosage and results of such drugs;
   e. Maintain a current list of qualified nurses on file.

---

sidered the most useful way to deal with procedures that are carried out by both professions [3].

A statement of this type regarding the role of nurses in intravenous therapy has been adopted in Massachusetts. Its text, which incorporates the rulings determined by the six organizations listed in Table 1, is presented in Table 2. As Anne Hargreaves [2] states, however:

It is important for each nurse to note that this policy statement will not provide immunity if the practitioner is negligent. The nurse should realize and be aware that any policy statement made by the professional organizations or by the employing agency does not relieve him/her of responsibility for his/her acts.

REFERENCES

1. Elman, R. Fluid balance from the nurse's point of view. *American Journal of Nursing* 49:222, 1949.
2. Hargreaves, A. Professional nurse practice committee. *Bulletin Massachusetts Nurses' Association,* Sept. 1965. P. 21.
3. Sward, K. M. (Staff consultant, American Nurses' Association). Personal communication, June 1967.
4. Williams, J. T., and Moravec, D. F. *Intravenous Therapy.* Hammond, Ind.: Clissold Publishing, 1967. Pp. 41–42.

2.
Intravenous Equipment

Vast improvements and innovations in intravenous equipment have increased the safety of infusion therapy. Newer equipment affords greater accuracy both in regulating the rate of flow and in controlling the volume, vital considerations in drug and electrolyte therapy. Disposable equipment has replaced the permanent rubber tubing administration sets. Pyrogenic reactions were more frequent following blood and fluid infusions through reused sets; these reactions were associated with improperly cleansed and unsterile equipment. The reusable sets required meticulous care in cleansing, rinsing, packing, and sterilizing by autoclave. The disposable unit, delivered sterile to the hospital, has saved patients from needless reactions.

Specialized equipment is available to meet every need of the patient. An understanding of this equipment is vital to the staff nurse, who shares the responsibility for safe fluid administration, and to the intravenous therapist, whose knowledge ensures the use of proper equipment.

Basic intravenous administration sets

The administration sets vary among manufacturing companies but are basically the same. An important factor is the rate of flow which the given set is gauged to produce; commercial sets vary—they may deliver from 10 to 25 drops per milliliter depending upon the nature of the fluid. Increased viscosity causes the size of the drop to increase so that a set that delivers 15 drops per milliliter will deliver 10 drops per milliliter when blood is administered. This information is of vital concern to the accurate control of the rate of infusion.

Pediatric sets

It is frequently necessary to maintain the flow at a minimum rate. One method is to reduce the size of the drop by the use of special sets, originally designed for pediatric infusions. These sets are valuable for use in parenteral therapy for the adult patient, since by reducing the size of the drop it is possible to maintain a constant intravenous flow with a minimum amount of fluid. These sets deliver 50 to 60 drops per milliliter, depending upon the viscosity of the solution; at the rate of 60 drops per minute it would take 1 hour to infuse 60 ml. Adapters are available (see Figure 1) for changing the flow rate of the regular set to 50 drops per milliliter. The adapter can easily be removed when an increase in the flow is desired.

Sets for monitoring infusion fluids

Sets are now available for measuring the amount of intravenous flow. Electronic meters allow a measured amount of solution to flow; the flow automatically stops when the required amount has been infused. A switch then triggers an alarm system which consists of a light at the nurses' station and a light and bell at the patient's bedside. Innovative varieties of such sets are being produced.

One set which monitors the patient's infusion fluids includes a small calibrated electrical switch attached to a hook from which the solution bottle hangs. When connected to a circuit containing a light or buzzer, this alert is calibrated to signal when the fluid level in the bottle drops to 50 ml. It can easily be calibrated to alarm at any desired level in order to give the nurse ample time to hang a new bottle before the intravenous container runs dry. This valuable device prevents patient dis-

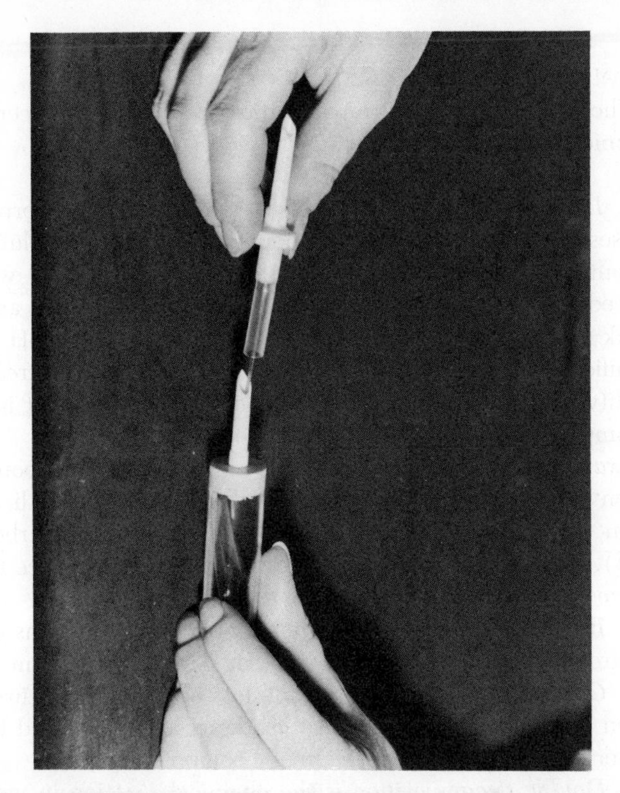

FIG. 1. Plexitron R38 M-50 administration set adapter for reducing drop size to $1/50$ ml inserted into drip chamber of administration set. This set will now deliver 50 drops per milliliter, enabling the patient to receive a slow infusion. (Travenol Laboratories, Inc., Morton Grove, Ill.)

comfort and preserves veins by avoiding the necessity of restarting the infusion.

A simple device has been manufactured which indicates the flow rate of the solution, both in drops per minute and in milliliters per hour (see Figure 2). It consists of a float chamber located between the two calibrations. The clamp is adjusted until a golden ball is suspended at the desired rate of flow. An

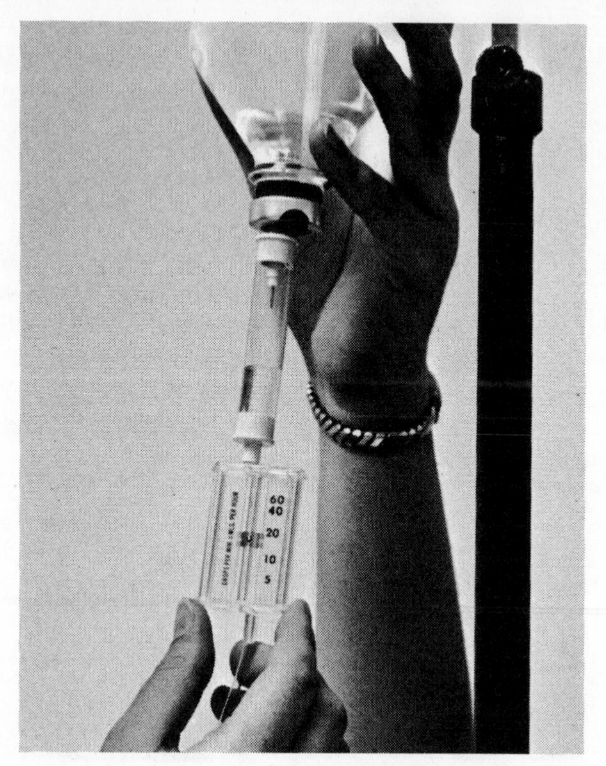

FIG. 2. I.V. Ometer indicates flow rate of the solution in drops per minute and milliliters per hour. (I.V. Ometer, Inc., Santa Cruz, Cal.)

added feature consists of a small red indicator which is slid over the prescribed rate of flow and alerts the nurse at a glance to any change in the flow. This set saves nursing time and is a valuable aid in maintaining the rate of flow of parenteral solutions.

MEDICATION SITES

Various devices are available for adding medications through the infusion needle or for setting up a secondary infusion. Some sets contain Y-type injection sites which facilitate this procedure. Twin-site supplementary sets are available (see Figure 3) for attaching to regular sets lacking these injection sites. Three-way stopcocks provide another method of introducing drugs through the infusion needle. These are especially valuable for anesthesia and for the operating room when supplementary medications are required, and when transfusions and secondary infusions are necessary.

Any opening into the tubing may permit air to be sucked into the infusion with danger of resultant air emboli. If three-

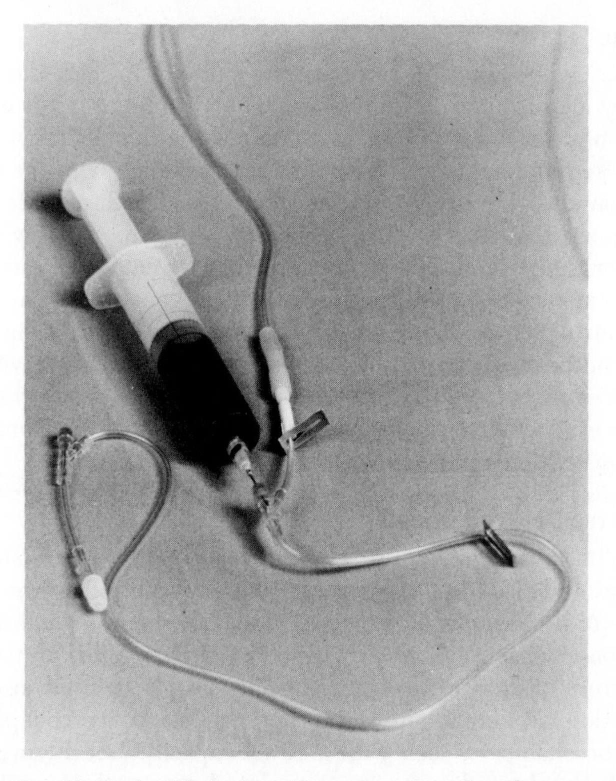

FIG. 3. Venotube Twin-Site Extension Set. Supplementary set containing Y-type injection sites. The needle is inserted directly through the medication site. (Dye added to facilitate photography.) (Abbott Laboratories, North Chicago, Ill.)

way stopcocks are used, caution must be exercised to see that the inlet not in use is completely shut off. The nurse should be alert for any faulty opening that allows air bubbles to escape into the flowing solution.

Medications can be added to solutions without interrupting the flow. In some solution bottles there is a site on the rubber bushing designed for this purpose. In certain types of administration sets, the air inlet in the set will accept the adapter of the syringe for introducing drugs.

Series hookup sets

Series hookup sets serve a useful purpose in fluid therapy. They allow fluid to be added or solutions to be changed while the infusion continues and also reduce the risk of solution containers running empty. Although these sets vary with the type of container used, the principle is the same. The disposable unit connects the two containers. The airvent in the primary container is closed and the secondary bottle is vented. The second container will empty first, but there may be a certain amount of mixing of fluids: if the specific gravity is greater in the second bottle there will be no mixing; if the specific gravity is greater in the primary container there will be some mixing. This is a factor to be considered in the use of solutions containing drugs that are incompatible.

Controlled volume sets

With the increasing use and number of solutions containing drugs and electrolytes, greater accuracy in controlling the volume of intravenous fluids is necessary. There are several innovations which permit accurate administration of measured volumes of fluids. One supplementary set, to be used in conjunction with an administration set, consists of five collapsible plastic chambers, each with a 10 ml capacity (see Figure 4). A clamp, depending on its placement between the chambers, controls the volume from 10 to 50 ml. This controlled volume set is particularly valuable when used as a secondary intravenous piggybacked through the medication site of the primary

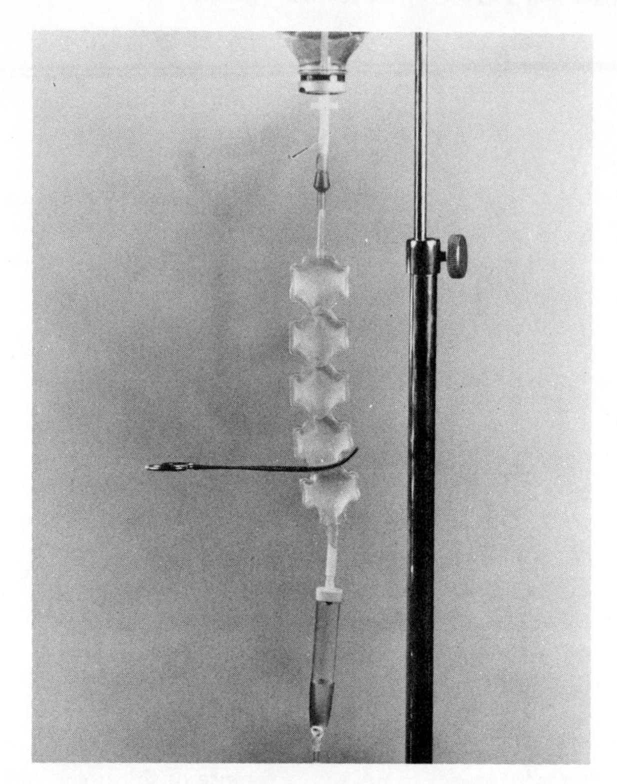

FIG. 4. The Pedatrol controls volume of intravenous fluids, permitting accurate administration of from 10 to 50 ml. (Travenol Laboratories, Inc., Morton Grove, Ill.)

infusion; measured volumes of solution containing drugs may then be administered on an intermittent basis. Such a set, with the clamp applied, is ventless, thus avoiding the risk that air may be introduced into the flowing solution once the chambers have emptied, a potential danger in some Y-type administration sets.

Other sets containing vented calibrated buret chambers control the volume to 100 ml (see Figure 5). The buret chamber of some sets contains a rubber float which prevents air from entering the tubing once the infusion is completed.

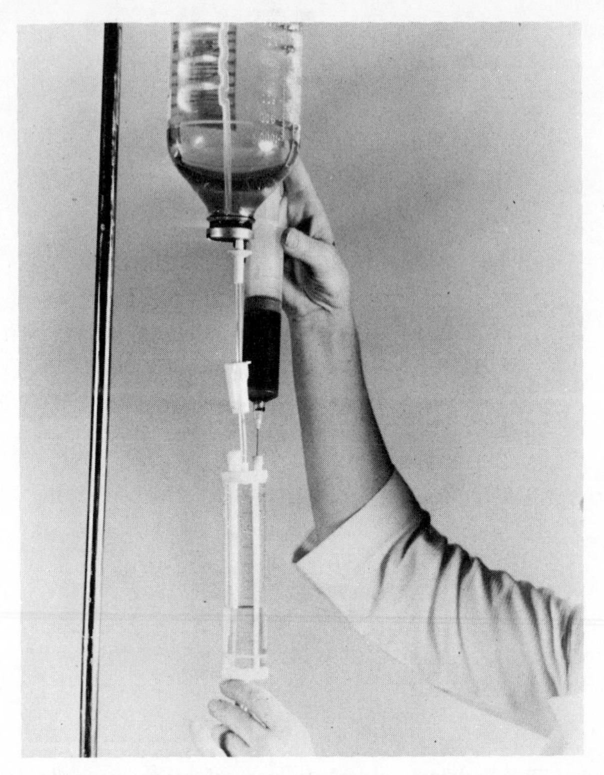

FIG. 5. Metriset. Calibrated chamber controls volume to 100 ml. Medications are added directly into the chamber through medication plug. (McGaw Laboratories, Inc., Glendale, Cal.; division of American Hospital Supply Corporation.)

Y-TYPE ADMINISTRATION SETS

A variety of commercial sets is available for alternate or simultaneous infusion of two solutions. Some sets contain a filter and a pressure unit for blood infusions.

There may be a significant hazard of air emboli when the Y-type administration set is used ignorantly or carelessly. Constant vigilance is necessary if both solutions are administered simultaneously. If one container is allowed to empty, large quantities of air can be sucked into the tubing; the empty bottle becomes the vent, due to the greater atmospheric pressure in the empty bottle and tube over the pressure below the partially constricted clamp in the tubing of the flowing solution [3].

Positive pressure sets

Positive pressure sets (see Figure 6) are designed to increase the rapidity of infusions and are an asset when rapid replace-

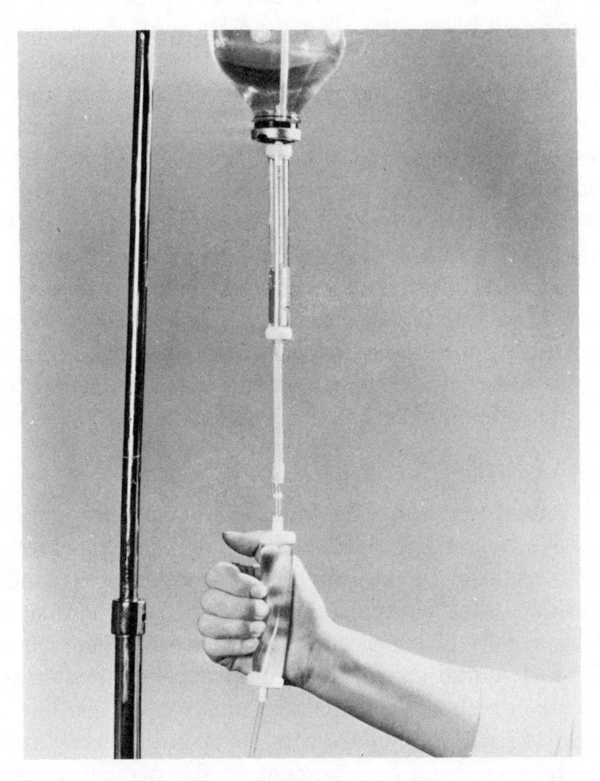

FIG. 6. Positive Pressure Set. Permits fluids to run by gravity with pressure unit available for rapid infusion should emergency arise. (McGaw Laboratories, Inc., Glendale, Cal.; division of American Hospital Supply Corporation.)

ment of fluid becomes necessary. They permit fluid to be administered by gravity, with a built-in pressure chamber available for rapid administration of blood should emergency arise. When used with the collapsible plastic blood unit, this system avoids the danger of air embolus; since the bag collapses, the need for air is eliminated. In contrast to the collapsible bag, the glass container must be vented to allow the fluid to flow; air pressure must be used when blood or fluid is forced into the blood stream. As the last portion of blood from the container is forced into the blood stream, the air under pressure may rapidly enter the vein before the clamp can be applied, resulting in a fatal embolus. According to Adriani [1], "Air pressure should not be used to force blood and other fluids into the blood stream."

The pump chamber must be filled at all times. The nurse should never apply positive pressure to infuse fluids; this is the responsibility of the physician.

The pressure cuff (see Figure 7) is another device which provides rapid infusion of blood. This cuff, with a pressure gauge calibrated in millimeters of mercury, fits over the plastic blood unit. Application of external pressure to the blood container permits rapid infusion of blood. This closed system avoids the inherent danger of air embolus.

Blood warmers

Prewarmed blood may be indicated when conditions (such as massive hemorrhage) exist that warrant large and rapid transfusions; cold blood administered under such conditions may produce effects of cardiac and general hypothermia. Boyan [2] cites results of observations carried out in the operating rooms of Memorial (Sloan-Kettering Cancer Center) Hospital, New York, which showed that the incidence of cardiac arrest during massive blood replacement (3000 milliliters or more per hour) dropped from 58.3 percent to 6.8 percent when cold bank blood was warmed to body temperature during infusion. He states: "To avoid the effects of cardiac and general hypo-

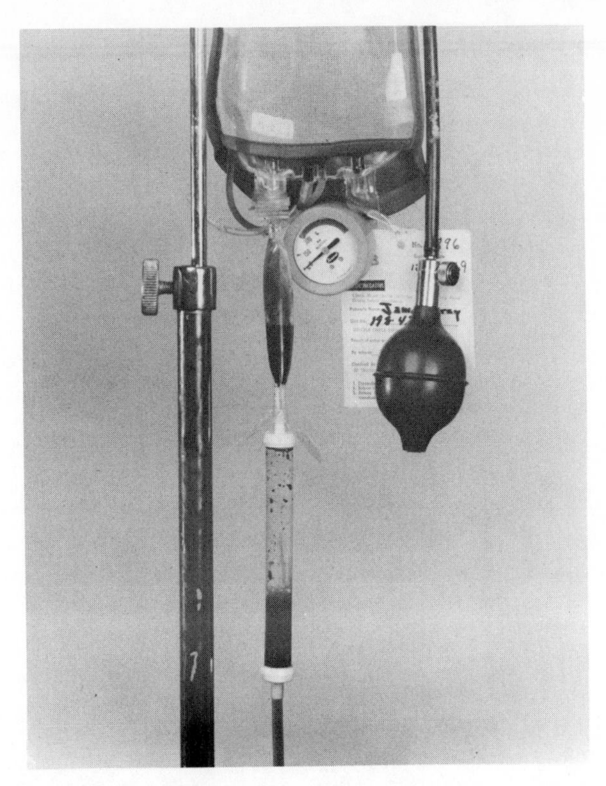

FIG. 7. Blood cuff, by means of external pressure, provides rapid infusion of blood. Inline filter is used. (Fenwal Laboratories, Morton Grove, Ill.; division of Travenol Laboratories, Inc.)

thermia during massive hemorrhage, cold bank blood should be warmed to body temperature when administered rapidly and in large amounts."

Several manufacturing companies have devised units consisting of blood-warming coils that are placed in warm water baths (see Figure 8). In one unit the blood is warmed at an approximate rate of 150 ml per minute in the adult coil and at approximately 50 ml per minute in the pediatric coil. Some

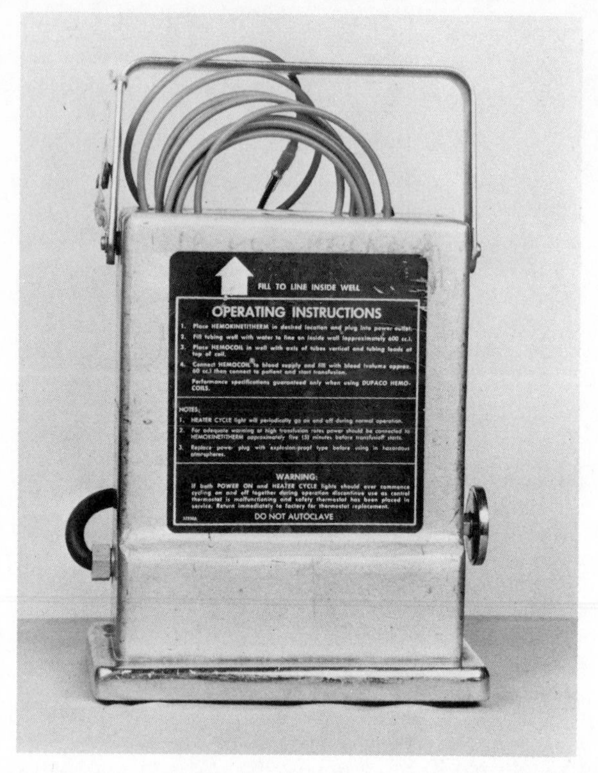

FIG. 8. Plexitron R66. Blood warmer with extension set. Extension coil with heating unit for administration of prewarmed blood. (Coil, Travenol Laboratories, Inc., Morton Grove, Ill.; heating unit, Hemokinetitherm Controlled Fluid Warmer, Dupaco Inc., Arcadia, Cal.)

units contain a water bath automatically controlled to maintain a desired temperature of between 39° C and 40° C, warming the blood to about 35° C.

Y-TYPE BLOOD COMPONENT SETS

Y-type blood component sets are available for the direct administration of platelets or cryoprecipitate (see Figure 9). One

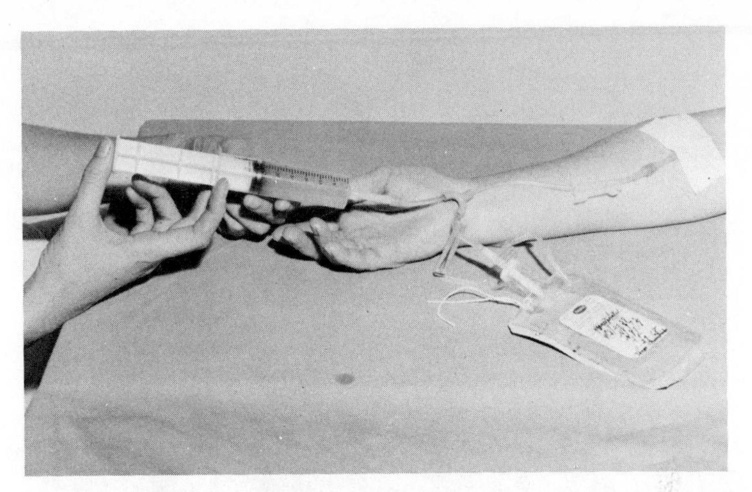

FIG. 9. Platelet Recipient Set. Platelets being infused through Y-type blood component set. (Fenwal Laboratories, Morton Grove, Ill.; division of Travenol Laboratories, Inc.)

arm of the Y contains a spike for introducing into the component bag; the other arm, an adapter for attaching a 50 cc syringe. The blood component is aspirated into the syringe; the main clamp is then opened, the air expelled, and the main line filled. A small mesh filter is enclosed within the adapter. The venipuncture is made and the component administered by syringe. The necessity for starting an initial infusion is eliminated and loss of components in the tubing is avoided.

Filter sets

A manufacturer has produced an administration set with a filter which blocks the passage of air and filters particulate matter to 0.45 microns (see Figure 10), a valuable device for infusing solutions with additives. It provides protection against possible precipitaton when used for administering hyperalimentation solutions. It eliminates the danger of air embolus when used with the electrical infusion pump. A wet filter with

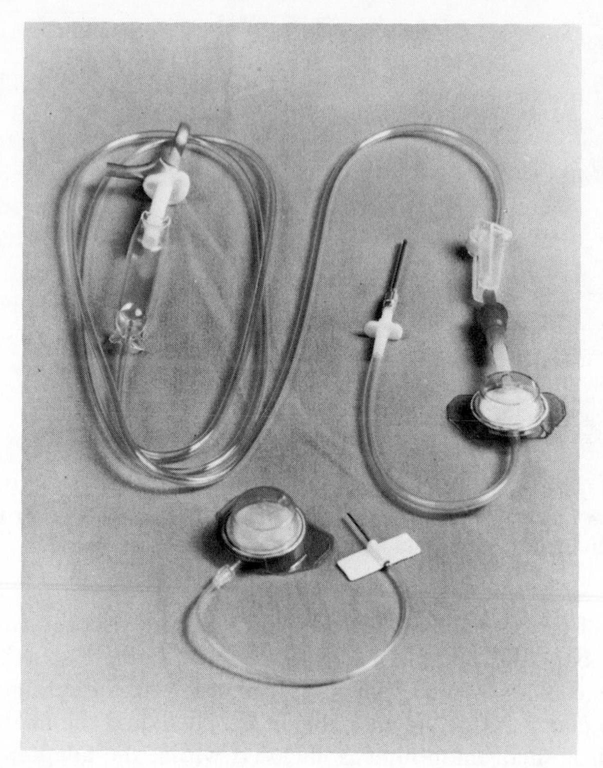

FIG. 10. Final Filter administration set containing a 0.45 micron porosity filter which, when wet, prevents passage of air as well as particulate matter. (Travenol Laboratories, Inc., Morton Grove, Ill.)

a 0.45 micron porosity connected between the pump and the patient prevents air from being pumped into the circulation should the infusion bottle become dry. Changing these sets every 24 hours prevents a potential build-up of bacteria in the filter. Blood administration sets with filters are available for the infusion of blood and blood components. Supplementary filters, for use in conjunction with administration sets, permit infusion of blood and afford easy replacement, preventing clogging when multiple bloods are infused.

ELECTRICAL INFUSION PUMPS

Electrical infusion pumps differ from the electronic meter sets in that they actually pump fluids at an exact predetermined rate, whereas the meter sets stop the flow when a measured amount of solution has been infused. As some may accurately pump as small an amount as 1 ml per hour, they assure safety in the administration of certain drugs, such as the vasopressors. They also provide safety in parenteral infusions. Because they maintain a constant rate of flow, they prevent the plugging of the needle that often occurs in infusions to small children when crying elevates the venous pressure and stops the flow. A charged battery permits cord-free operation when transportation of the patient is necessary.

REFERENCES

1. Adriani, J. Venipuncture. *American Journal of Nursing* 62:70, 1962.
2. Boyan, C. P. Cold or warmed blood for massive transfusion. *Annals of Surgery* 160:282, 1964.
3. Tarail, R. Practice of fluid therapy. *Journal of the American Medical Association* 171:45–49, 1950.

3.

Anatomy and Physiology Applied to Intravenous Therapy

Intravascular therapy consists of the introduction of fluids, blood, and drugs directly into the vascular system; that is, into arteries, into bone marrow, and into veins. The usual reason for using the *intra-arterial route* is to introduce radiopaque material for diagnostic purposes such as arteriograms for cerebral disorders. The dangers of arterial spasm and subsequent gangrene present problems which make this type of therapy hazardous for therapeutic use [2]. The *bone marrow,* because of its venous plexus, can be utilized for intravascular therapy. However, because infusions into the bone marrow can be dangerous, this route should be used only if other channels are unavailable. Repeated intramarrow injections could result in osteomyelitis. The *veins,* because of their abundance and location, present the most readily accessible route.

Applied to intravascular therapy, knowledge of the anatomy and physiology of veins and arteries is essential to the proficiency of the therapist and the welfare of the patient. Through a study of the superficial veins the therapist acquires a sense of discrimination in the choice of veins for intravenous use. Many factors must be considered in selecting a vein; the anatomical characteristics offer a basis for good judgment. The size, location, and resilience of the vein affect its desirability for infusion purposes.

Familiarity with the principles underlying venous physiology is also of prime value to the therapist. An understanding of the reaction of veins to the nervous stimulation of the vasoconstrictors and vasodilators enables the therapist to (1) increase the size and visibility of a vein before attempting venipuncture, and (2) relieve venous spasm and thus assist in infusion maintenance.

With proficiency of the therapist, the primary goal of intravenous therapy is achieved: the welfare of the patient. Painless and effective therapy is desirable, promoting the patient's comfort and well-being, and often his complete recovery from disease or trauma as well. An integral part of this goal is the recognition and prevention of complications. The therapist, through her knowledge of anatomy and physiology, can reduce these risks.

Phlebitis and *thrombosis* are by far the commonest complications resulting from parenteral therapy. Although seemingly mild, they do present serious consequences: they (1) cause moderate to severe discomfort, often taking many days or weeks to subside, and (2) limit the available veins for further therapy. Injury to the endothelial lining of the vein contributes to these local complications. A thorough understanding of the peripheral veins alerts the therapist to observe precautions in technique in performing venipunctures. Proper technique in venipuncture minimizes the trauma to the vessel wall and provides an entry as painless and safe as possible. Examination of the superficial veins of the lower extremities alerts the therapist to the dangers resulting from their use. By avoiding venipunctures in veins prone to varicosities and sluggish circulation, the likelihood of phlebitis and thrombosis is decreased and the secondary risk of *pulmonary embolism* is reduced.

Awareness of the characteristics that differentiate veins from arteries assists the therapist in reducing the risk of *necrosis* and *gangrene*; these serious complications occur when a medication is injected into an artery as the result of an inadvertent arterial puncture.

An understanding of the anatomy and physiology of the veins

and arteries enables the therapist to recognize the existence of an *arteriovenous anastomosis;* failure to recognize this condition results in repeated and unsuccessful venipunctures performed in an attempt to initiate the infusion. These repeated punctures compound the trauma to the inner lining of the vein and increase the risk of the local complications already described, any of which limits the number of available veins, interrupts the course of therapy, and causes unnecessary pain and even dire consequence for the patient.

VASCULAR SYSTEM

The circulatory system of the body is divided into two main systems, the pulmonary and the systemic, each with its own set of vessels. The *pulmonary system* consists of the blood flow from the right ventricle of the heart to the lungs, where it is oxygenated and returned to the left atrium. The *systemic system,* the larger of the two, is the one which concerns the intravenous therapist. It consists of the aorta, arteries, arterioles, capillaries, venules, and veins through which the blood must flow. The blood leaves the left ventricle, flows to all parts of the body, and returns to the right atrium of the heart via the vena cava. The *systemic veins* are divided into three classes: (1) superficial, (2) deep, and (3) venous sinuses [3].

Superficial veins

The superficial or cutaneous veins are those used in venipuncture. They are located just beneath the skin in the superficial fascia. These veins and the deep veins sometimes unite; in the lower extremities they unite freely [4]. For example, the small saphenous vein, a superficial vein, drains the dorsum of the foot and the posterior section of the leg; it ascends the back of the leg and empties directly into the deep popliteal vein. Before the small saphenous vein terminates in the deep popliteal, it sends out a branch which, after joining the great saphenous vein, also terminates in a deep vein, the femoral vein. Because of these deep connections, great concern arises when it becomes necessary to use the veins in the lower extremities. A thrombosis may occur which could easily extend to the deep veins and cause pulmonary embolism [2]. Understanding this, the nurse should refrain from the use of these veins.

Varicosities occurring in the lower extremities, although readily available to venipuncture, are not a satisfactory route for parenteral administration. The relatively stagnant blood in such veins is prone to clot, resulting in a superficial phlebitis. Medication injected below a varicosity may result in another potential danger, a collection of the infused drug in the varicosity. This is caused by the stagnant blood flow. This "pocket" of infused medication may delay the effect of the drug when immediate action is desired; another concern is the danger of untoward reactions to the drug which may occur when this accumulation reaches the general circulation [1].

Arteriovenous anastomosis

Deep veins are usually enclosed in the same sheath with the arteries. Occasionally an arteriovenous anastomosis may occur on a congenital basis or as the result of past penetrating injury of the vein and adjacent artery. When such trauma occurs, the blood flows directly from the artery into the vein; as a result the veins, draining an arteriovenous fistula, are overburdened with high pressure arterial blood. These veins appear large and tortuous. In these unusual circumstances the therapist's quick recognition of an arteriovenous fistula may prevent pain, complications, and loss of time, due to repeated unsuccessful attempts to start the infusion.

Arteries and veins

Knowledge of the characteristics differentiating veins from arteries and the position of each is important to the therapist so that she may avoid the complications of an inadvertent arterial puncture. Arteries and veins are similar in structure; both are composed of three layers of tissue. A close examination of these layers reveals their differing characteristics.

1. *Tunica intima* or *inner layer* consists of an inner elastic endothelial lining which also forms the valves in veins. These valves are absent in arteries. The endothelial lining is identical in the arteries and the veins, consisting of a smooth layer of flat cells. This smooth surface allows the cells and platelets to flow through the blood vessels without interruption under normal conditions. Care must be taken to avoid roughening this surface when performing a venipuncture or removing a needle from a vein. Any trauma which roughens the endothelial lining encourages the process of thrombosis whereby cells and platelets adhere to the vessel wall [2].

Many veins contain valves which are semilunar folds of the endothelium. These valves are found in the larger veins of the extremities; their function is to keep the blood flowing toward the heart. Where muscular pressure would cause a backing up of the blood supply, these valves play an important role. They occur at points of branching and often cause a noticeable bulge in the veins. Applying a tourniquet to the extremity impedes the venous flow. When suction is applied, as occurs in the process of drawing blood, the valves compress and close the lumen of the vein, preventing the backward flow of the blood. These valves thus interfere with the process of withdrawing blood. Recognizing the presence of a valve, the nurse may resolve the difficulty by slightly readjusting the needle.

These valves are absent in many of the small veins, which can therefore be utilized when, due to obstruction from a thrombosis in the ascending vein, they would otherwise prove useless. The needle may be inserted below the thrombosis with its direction toward the distal end of the extremity; this results in a rerouting of the fluid and avoidance of the thrombosed portion.

2. *Tunica media* or *middle layer* consists of muscular and elastic tissue. The nerve fibers, both vasoconstrictors and vasodilators, are located in this middle layer. These fibers, constantly receiving impulses from the vasoconstrictor center in the medulla, keep the vessels in a state of tonus. They also stimulate both arteries and veins to contract or relax. The middle

layer is not as strong and stiff in the veins as in the arteries, and therefore the veins tend to collapse or distend as the pressure within falls or rises. Arteries do not collapse.

Stimulation by a change in temperature or by mechanical or chemical irritation may produce spasms in the vein or artery. For instance, interrupting a continuous infusion to administer a pint of cold blood may produce vasoconstriction; this results in spasm, impedes the flow of blood, and causes pain. Application of heat to the vein promotes vasodilation, which will relieve the spasm, improve the flow of blood, and relieve the pain. The same results are obtained by heat when an irritating drug has caused vasoconstriction. In this situation, heat serves a twofold purpose: it (1) relieves the spasm and increases the blood flow, and (2) protects the vessel wall from inflammation caused by the medication—with heat dilating the vein and increasing the flow of blood, the drug becomes more diluted and less irritating. The use of heat to achieve vasodilation is also an aid when it becomes necessary to use veins that are small and poorly filled.

Spasms produced by a chemical irritation in an artery may result in dire consequence. A single artery supplies circulation to a particular area. If this artery is damaged, the related area will suffer from impaired circulation and possibly from necrosis and gangrene. If a chemical agent is introduced into the artery, a spasm may result—a contraction that could shut off the blood supply completely. This problem is not as serious when veins are used, since many veins supply a particular area; if one is injured, others will maintain the circulation.

3. *Tunica adventitia* or *outer layer* consists of areolar connective tissue; it surrounds and supports the vessel. In arteries this layer is thicker than in veins because it is subjected to greater pressure from the force of blood within.

Arteries need more protection than veins and are so placed that injury is less likely to occur. Whereas veins are superficially located, most arteries lie deep in the tissues and are protected by muscle. Occasionally an artery is located superficially in an unusual place; this artery is then called an *aberrant artery*. An aberrant artery must not be mistaken for a vein. If a chemical which causes spasm is introduced into an aberrant artery, permanent damage may result [2].

Arteries pulsate and veins do not, a helpful differentiating characteristic.

Superficial veins of the upper extremities

The superficial veins of the upper extremities are shown in Figures 11 and 12. They consist of the following: digital, metacarpal, cephalic, basilic, and median veins.

DIGITAL VEINS. The dorsal digital veins flow along the lateral portions of the fingers and are joined to each other by communicating branches [3]. At times these veins are available as a last resort for fluid administration. In some patients they are prominent enough to accommodate a 21-gauge scalp vein needle. With adequate taping the fingers can be completely immobilized, thereby preventing the needle from puncturing the posterior wall of the vein and causing extravasation of fluid.

METACARPAL VEINS. The three metacarpal veins are formed by the union of the digital veins [3]. The position of these veins makes them well adapted for intravenous use; the needle and adapter, in most cases, lie flat between the joints and the metacarpal bones of the hand, the bones themselves providing a natural splint. The early use of the metacarpal veins is important in a course of parenteral therapy. Irritating fluid passing through a vein traumatized by previous puncture causes inflammation and pain. Therefore performing venipunctures for fluid administration at the distal end of the extremity, early in the course of therapy, is beneficial; it enables the nurse to initiate each successive venipuncture above the previous puncture site. Unnecessary inflammation and pain are avoided and opportunity for multiple venipunctures is provided.

Occasionally the use of the metacarpal veins in the elderly is contraindicated. Due to inadequate tissue and thin skin in

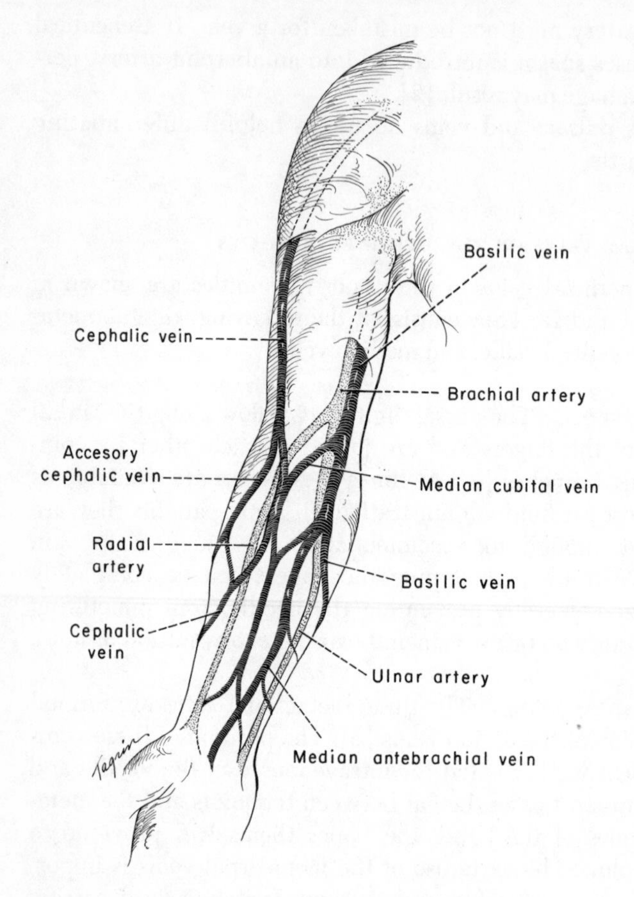

FIG. 11. Superficial veins of the forearm.

this area, extravasation of blood on venipuncture may readily occur.

CEPHALIC VEIN. The cephalic vein has its source in the radial part of the dorsal venous network formed by the metacarpal veins. Receiving tributaries from both surfaces of the forearm,

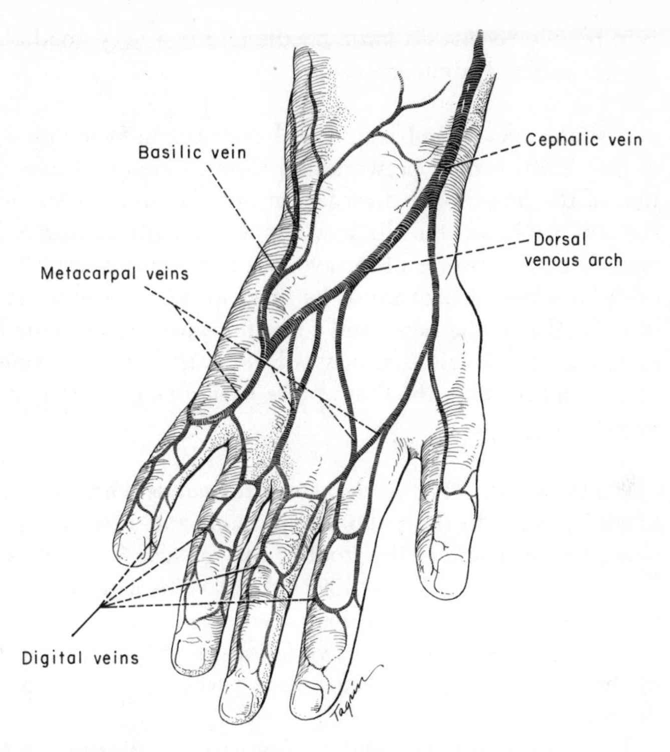

FIG. 12. Superficial veins of the dorsal aspect of the hand.

it flows upward along the radial border of the forearm [3]. Because of its size and position, this vein provides an excellent route for transfusion administration. It readily accommodates a large needle and, by nature of its position in the forearm, a natural splinting is provided for the needle and adapter.

The *accessory cephalic vein* originates from either one of two sources: a plexus on the back of the forearm or the dorsal venous network. Ascending the arm, it joins the cephalic vein below the elbow. Occasionally it arises from that portion of the cephalic vein just above the wrist and flows back into the main cephalic vein at some higher point [3]. The accessory cephalic vein readily receives a large needle and is a very good choice for use in blood administration.

BASILIC VEIN. The basilic vein has its origin in the ulna part of the dorsal venous network and ascends along the ulna portion of the forearm. It diverges toward the anterior surface of the arm just below the elbow where it meets the median cubital vein. During a course of intravenous therapy this large vein is often overlooked because of its inconspicuous position on the ulna border of the hand and forearm; when other veins have been exhausted, this vein may still be available. By flexing the elbow and bending the arm up the basilic vein is brought into view.

MEDIAN VEINS. The *median antebrachial vein* arises from the venous plexus on the palm of the hand and extends upward along the ulna side of the front of the forearm; it empties into the basilic vein or the median cubital vein. This vein, when prominent, affords a route for parenteral fluid administration. However, there are frequent variations of the superficial veins of the forearm, and this vein is not always present as a well-defined vessel.

The *median cephalic* and *median basilic veins* in the antecubital fossa are the veins most generally used for withdrawal of blood. Because of their size and superficial location, they are readily accessible for venipuncture. They receive a large size needle and, due to the muscular and connective tissue supporting them, have little tendency to roll.

Since the median cephalic vein crosses in front of the brachial artery, care must be taken during venipuncture to avoid puncturing the artery. Accidential intra-arterial injection of a drug could result in permanent damage.

The basilic vein, outside the antecubital fossa on the ulna curve of the arm, is the least desirable for venipuncture. On removal of the needle a hematoma may readily occur if the patient flexes his elbow to stop the bleeding rather than elevating the arm in the preferred manner.

THE SKIN

The skin is made up of two layers, the epidermis and the dermis. The *epidermis* is the uppermost layer which forms a protective covering for the dermis. Its degree of thickness varies in different parts of the body. It is thickest on the palms of the hands and the soles of the feet and thinnest on the inner surface of the limbs. Its degree of thickness also varies with age. In an elderly patient the skin on the dorsum of the hand may be so thin that it does not adequately support the vein for venipuncture when parenteral infusions are required.

The *dermis* or underlayer is highly sensitive and vascular. It contains many capillaries and thousands of nerve fibers. These nerve fibers are of different types and include those which react to temperature, touch, pressure, and pain. The number of nerve fibers varies in different areas of the body. Some areas of the body skin are highly sensitive; other areas are only mildly sensitive. The insertion of a needle in one area may cause a great deal of pain, while another area may be practically painless. In our experience the inner aspect of the wrist is a highly sensitive area. Venipunctures are performed here only when other veins have been exhausted.

SUPERFICIAL FASCIA

The superficial fascia, or subcutaneous areolar connective tissue, lies below the two layers of skin and is, in itself, another covering. It is in this fascia that the superficial veins are located. It varies in thickness. When a needle is inserted into this fascia, there is free movement of the skin above. Great care in aseptic technique must be observed, as an infection in this loose tissue spreads easily. Such an infection is called *cellulitis* [4].

REFERENCES

1. Abbott Laboratories. Entering the Vein. *Parenteral Administration.* North Chicago, Ill., 1959. P. 6.

2. Adriani, J. Venipuncture. *American Journal of Nursing* 62:66–69, 1962.
3. Goss, C. M. (ed.). *Gray's Anatomy of the Human Body* (27th ed.). Philadelphia: Lea & Febiger, 1965. Pp. 742–744.
4. Kimber, D. C., Gray, C. E., and Stackpoles, C. E. *Textbook of Anatomy and Physiology* (15th ed.). New York: Macmillan, 1966. Pp. 69, 398, 423–431.

4.
Technique of Intravenous Therapy

APPROACH TO THE PATIENT

The manner with which the nurse approaches the patient may have a direct bearing on his response to intravenous therapy. Since an undesirable response can affect his ability to accept treatment, emphasis must be placed on the significance of the nurse's manner and approach.

Intravenous therapy, though routine to the nurse, may be a new and frightening experience to the patient who is unfamiliar with the procedure. He may have heard rumors of fatalities associated with infusions or may misinterpret the treatment. By explaining the procedure to the patient, the nurse will alleviate his fears and help him to accept therapy.

The critically ill patient is particularly prone to fears which can at times become exaggerated, triggering an undesirable autonomic nervous system response usually known as a vasovagal reaction. Such a reaction may manifest itself in the form of syncope and can be prevented if the nurse appears confident and reassures the patient. Sympathetic reaction may follow syncope and result in vasoconstriction. Peripheral collapse then limits available veins, complicating the venipuncture. Repeated attempts at venipuncture can result in an experience so traumatic as to affect the further course of fluid therapy. Only a skilled person should perform a venipuncture on an anxious patient with limited and difficult veins.

Reactions to exaggerated fear may not only make therapy difficult, but may constitute a real threat to the severe cardiac patient. Welt [7] has illustrated such a reaction in a case of pulmonary edema in a patient with renal insufficiency and hypertensive and arteriosclerotic heart disease with failure. No explanation of the infusion was made to the patient. When the needle was inserted, acute pulmonary edema occurred. The intravenous was discontinued and in a few hours the patient recovered. Later that day, after the procedure was explained and the patient was sedated, 1000 ml of whole blood was tolerated. We can easily visualize such a reaction when we review the body's response to stress. Fear incites stimulation of the adrenal medulla to secrete the vasopressors which help maintain blood pressure and increase the work of the heart. Increased adrenal cortical secretions result in (1) sodium and chloride retention, which causes water retention, and (2) loss of cellular potassium, which draws water with it into the intravascular system. Increased antidiuretic hormone secretions cause a decreased urinary output, which results in retention of fluids and an increase in blood volume [4]. Such an increase may be sufficient to send a patient with an overburdened vascular system into pulmonary edema.

SELECTING THE VEIN

The selection of the vein may be a deciding factor in the success of the infusion and in the preservation of veins for future therapy. The most prominent vein is not necessarily the most suitable for venipuncture: prominence may be due to a sclerosed condition which occludes the lumen and interferes with the flow of solution; or the prominent vein may be located in an area impractical for infusion purposes [2]. Scrutiny of the veins in both arms is desirable before a choice is made. The prime factors to be considered in selecting a vein are (1) suitable location, (2) condition of the vein, (3) purpose of the infusion, and (4) duration of therapy.

LOCATION

Most superficial veins are accessible for venipuncture, but some of these veins, because of their location, are not practical. The *antecubital veins* are such veins, located over an area of joint flexion where any motion could dislodge the needle and cause infiltration or result in a mechanical phlebitis. If these large veins are impaired or damaged a phlebothrombosis may occur which could limit the many available hand veins. The antecubital veins offer excellent sources for withdrawing blood and may be used numerous times without damage to the vein, provided good technique and sharp needles are used. But one infusion of long duration may traumatize the vein, limiting these vessels which most readily provide ample quantities of blood when large samples are needed.

Because of the close proximity of the arteries to the veins in the antecubital fossa, special care must be observed to prevent intra-arterial injection when medications are introduced. An artery can generally be detected by the thicker and tougher wall, the brighter red blood, and usually the presence of a pulse. *Aberrant arteries* in the antecubital area have been found to exist in one person out of ten. When a patient complains of severe pain in the hand or arm upon infusion, an arteriospasm due to an intra-arterial injection is to be suspected and the infusion must be stopped immediately.

Surgery often dictates which extremity is to be used. Veins should be avoided in the affected arm of an axillary dissection, such as a radical mastectomy; the circulation may be embarrassed, affecting the flow of the infusion and increasing the edema. When the patient is turned on his side during the operation the upper arm is used for the intravenous; increased venous pressure in the lower arm may interfere with the free flow of the solution.

Objection is frequently expressed to the use of the veins in the lower extremities. As stated in Chapter 2, these objections arise from the danger of a pulmonary embolism due to a thrombosis extending into the deep veins. Complications may also arise from the stagnant blood in varicosities; pooling of infused medications can cause untoward reactions when a toxic concentration reaches the circulating blood. Varicosities, because of the stagnant blood, are prone to trauma. Phlebitis interferes with ambulation of the patient.

Condition of the vein

Frequently the dorsal metacarpal veins provide points of entry that should be utilized first in order to preserve the proximal veins for further therapy. The use of these veins depends upon their condition. In some elderly patients, the dorsal metacarpal veins may be a poor choice; blood extravasation occurs more readily in small thin veins, and difficulty may be encountered in adequately securing the needle because of thin skin and lack of supportive tissue. At times these veins do not dilate sufficiently to allow for successful venipuncture; when hypovolemia occurs the peripheral veins collapse quicker than do the large ones.

Palpation of the vein is an important step in determining the condition of the vein and in differentiating it from a pulsating artery. A thrombosed vein may be detected by its lack of resilience, by its hard, cord-like feeling, and by the ease with which it rolls. Use of such traumatized veins can only result in repeated venipunctures, pain, and undue stress.

Occasionally when thrombosis from multiple infusions interferes with the flow of solution and limits available veins, the venipuncture may be performed with the needle inserted in the direction of the distal end; lack of valves in these small peripheral veins permits rerouting of the solution and a bypassing of the involved vein.

Often large veins may be detected by palpation and offer advantage over the smaller but more readily discernible veins. Due to the small blood volume, the more superficial veins may not be easily palpated and may not make a satisfactory choice for venipuncture.

Continual use by the nurse of the same fingers for palpation will increase their sensitivity. The thumb should never be used since it is not as sensitive as the fingers; also a pulse may be detected in the nurse's thumb, and this may be confused with an aberrant artery.

Although not apparent, edema may conceal an available vein; pressure for a few seconds with the fingers often helps to disperse the fluid and define the vein.

Purpose of the infusion

The purpose of the infusion dictates the rate of flow and the solution to be infused—two factors which inherently affect the selection of the vein. When large quantities of fluid are to be rapidly infused, or when positive pressure is indicated, a large vein must be used. When fluids with a high viscosity such as packed cells are required, a vein with an adequate blood volume is necessary to ensure flow of the solution.

Large veins are used when hypertonic solutions or solutions containing irritating drugs are to be infused. Such solutions traumatize small veins; the supply of blood in these veins is not sufficient to dilute the infused fluid.

Duration of therapy

A prolonged course of therapy requires multiple infusions which makes preservation of the veins essential. Performing the venipuncture distally with each subsequent puncture proximal to the previous one and alternating arms will contribute to this preservation.

The patient's comfort is also a factor that should be considered when infusions are required over an extended period of time; avoiding areas over joint flexion and performing venipunctures on veins located on the dorsal surface of the extremities will provide more freedom and comfort to the patient.

SELECTING THE NEEDLE

Infusion may be administered through a catheter or metal needle.

Three types of catheter are available (see Figure 13):

1. *Plastic needle* (catheter mounted on a needle). Once the venipuncture is made, the catheter is slipped off the needle into the vein and the metal needle removed. Plastic stylets are available for inserting into the catheter to maintain patency for intermittent infusion.
2. *Intracatheter* (catheter inserted through the needle). The venipuncture is performed, the catheter is then pushed through the needle until the desired length is within the lumen of the vein, and the cutting edge is protected by a shield to prevent the catheter from being severed.
3. *Inlying catheter.* This catheter is inserted by means of a minor surgical procedure (cut-down) performed by the physician.

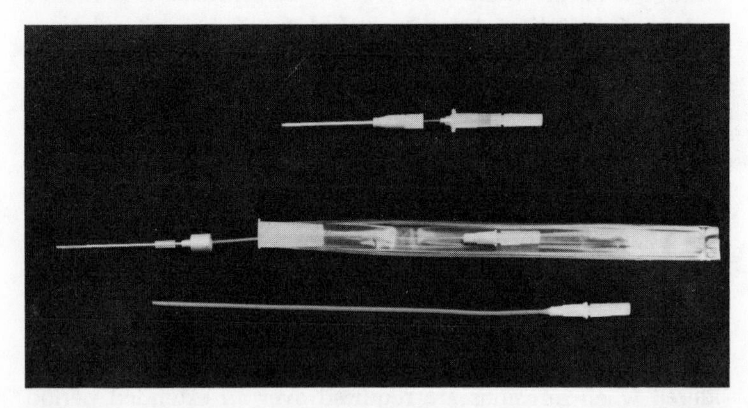

FIG. 13. Three types of intravenous catheter. (*Top*) Plastic needle. (Deseret Angiocath.) (*Center*) Intracatheter. (Deseret Intracath.) (*Bottom*) Inlying catheter inserted through a cut-down. (Deseret Cut-Down Catheter.) (Deseret Pharmaceutical Co., Sandy, Utah.)

The choice of catheter depends upon the purpose of the infusion, and the condition and availability of the veins.

Plastic needles are used in the operating room to ensure a ready route for the administration of blood, and fluid. In long-term therapy the plastic needle serves a purpose when difficulty arises in keeping the needle in the vein.

The intracatheter is used when a longer catheter is desired. It affords less risk of infiltration than the metal needle, often being used for administering drugs or hypertonic solutions which may cause necrosis if extravasation occurs.

An inlying catheter is required when (1) veins become exhausted from prolonged therapy, (2) obesity obscures the veins, and (3) peripheral veins have collapsed from shock.

Most catheters are siliconized for easy insertion and radiopaque for x-ray detection.

Metal needles are usually used for infusions of short duration. Two types are available: the scalp vein needle and the commonly used straight needle.

The *scalp vein needle* is approximately ¾ of an inch long and ranges in size from a 23-gauge bore to a 16-gauge bore. This needle was originally designed for pediatric and geriatric use and is now useful in prolonged therapy for all ages. It has three definite advantages: (1) the thin wall offers a large lumen with a smaller needle diameter, (2) the short bevel reduces the risk of infiltration from puncture to the wall of the vein, and (3) the plastic wings, used for holding the needle while performing the venipuncture, fold flat against the skin affording better anchoring power than the straight needle with a bulky hub.

The factors to be considered in selecting a metal needle are: length of bevel, gauge, and length of the needle.

A short *bevel* reduces the risk of (1) trauma to the endothelial wall, (2) infiltration from a puncture to the posterior wall, and (3) hematoma or extravasation occurring when the needle enters the vein. When a needle with a long bevel is inserted into the vessel, blood may leak into the tissues before the entire bevel is within the lumen of the vein.

Whenever possible the *gauge of the needle* should be appreciably smaller than the lumen of the vein to be entered; with the gauge of the needle approaching the size of the vein, trauma may occur. When a large needle occludes the flow of blood, irritating solutions flowing through the vein, with no dilution of blood, may cause a chemical phlebitis. A mechanical phlebitis may result from motion and pressure exerted by the needle on the endothelial wall of the vein.

When large amounts of fluid are required, a needle of adequate size must be used; a small lumen interferes with the flow of solution. As Adriani [2] states, "The flow of blood varies inversely as the fourth power of the radius of the lumen of the needle. Thus, a needle with an internal radius of 1 mm. delivering 1 cc. of blood with a fixed pressure on the plunger or in the infusion bottle delivers only 1/16 of a cc. when the radius is reduced to ½ mm." A large needle is also required with fluids of high viscosity. The rate of flow of the solution decreases in proportion to the viscosity of the fluid.

The flow of the solution varies inversely with the *length of the needle shaft.* If the length of the needle is increased, other conditions being equal, the volume flowing will be reduced [2]. Use of a short needle for infusions reduces the risk of infiltration. Because a long needle affords less play than a short needle, less motion is needed to puncture the vessel wall.

SECURING PROPER LIGHTING

The importance of proper lighting should not be overlooked. A few extra seconds spent in obtaining adequate light may actually save time and free the patient from unnecessary venipunctures. The ideal light is either an ample amount of daylight or a spotlight which does not shine directly on the vein, but which leaves enough shadow for clearly defining the vessel.

APPLYING THE TOURNIQUET

Special care must be taken to distend the vein adequately. To achieve this, a soft rubber tourniquet is applied with enough pressure to impede the venous flow while the arterial flow is maintained; if the radial pulse cannot be felt the tourniquet is too tight. In order to fill the veins to capacity, pressure is applied until radial pulsation ceases, and then released until pulsation begins. A blood pressure cuff may be used; inflate the cuff and then release it until the pressure drops to just below the diastolic pressure.

The tourniquet is applied to the mid-forearm if the selected vein is in the dorsum of the hand. If the selected vein is in the forearm, the tourniquet is applied to the upper arm.

Very little pressure is applied when performing venipunctures on patients with sclerosed veins. If the pressure is too great or the tourniquet is left on for an extended length of time the vein will become hard and tortuous, causing added difficulty when the needle is introduced. For some sclerosed veins a tourniquet is unnecessary and only makes the phlebotomy more difficult.

If pressure exerted by the tourniquet does not fill the veins sufficiently, the patient may be asked to open and close his fist. The action of the muscles will force the blood into the veins causing them to distend considerably more. Frequently a light tapping will help fill the vein. Occasionally these methods are inadequate to fill the vein sufficiently. In such cases application of heat is helpful. To be effective the heat must be applied to the entire extremity for 10 to 20 minutes and retained until the venipuncture is performed.

PREPARATION FOR VENIPUNCTURE

The equipment is assembled and the solution is carefully examined for any change in appearance or for the presence of particulate matter. The label should be checked to ensure it is the appropriate solution. The tubing is then attached to the bottle and the drip chamber filled to expedite clearing the infusion set of air by preventing air bubbles from entering the tubing.

The patient should be in a comfortable position with his arm on a flat surface. If necessary a strip of tape is used to secure the arm to an armboard and prevent an uncooperative or disoriented patient from jerking his arm while the needle is being inserted.

If the area selected for venipuncture is hairy, shaving will permit better cleansing of the skin and make removal of the needle less painful when the infusion is terminated.

TECHNIQUES IN VENIPUNCTURE

Direct method or stab technique

This method is performed with a thrust of the needle through the skin and into the vein with one quick motion. The needle enters the skin directly over the vein. This technique is excellent as long as large veins are available. Due to the many times one must resort to the use of small veins, this is not the preferred technique. Such an attempt at entry into the small veins will result in hematomas. If the nurse chooses to use this technique she will never be adept at phlebotomies on tiny venules when the situation arises.

Indirect method

This method consists of two complete motions:

1. Insertion of the needle through the skin. The needle enters the skin below the point where the vein is visible; entering the skin above the vein tends to depress the vein, obscuring its position.
2. Relocation of the vein and entry into the vein.

BASIC VENIPUNCTURE

The basic venipuncture is performed as follows (see Figure 14):

1. Apply tourniquet and select vein.

2. Prepare skin with an accepted antiseptic—70 percent isopropanol is usually used.

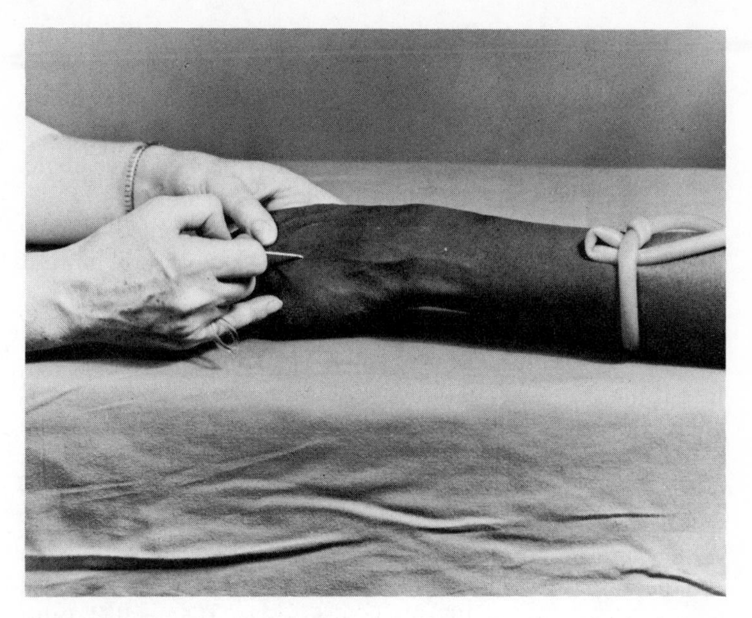

FIG. 14. Infusion tubing kinked between third and little fingers. Left thumb keeps skin taut and anchors vein. The needle is held in line with the vein at 45° angle.

3. After establishing a minimum rate of flow by adjusting the clamp, kink the infusion tubing between the third and little fingers of the right hand. When the kinked tubing is released, the minimum rate of flow will prevent a rapid infusion of fluid and drugs with the potential danger of speed shock. Obstructing flow of solution manually expedites the procedure and leaves hands free for anchoring the needle and caring for any collected blood samples.

4. Hold the patient's hand or arm with the left hand, using the thumb to keep the skin taut and to anchor the vein to prevent rolling.

5. Place the needle in line with the vein, about one half inch below proposed site of entry. The bevel-up position of the needle facilitates venipuncture and produces less trauma to the skin and the vein on puncture.

In small veins it is often necessary to enter the vein with the bevel down to prevent extravasation; any readjustment of the needle should be made before releasing the tourniquet to prevent puncturing the vein and producing a hematoma [1].

6. Insert needle through skin and tissue at a 45 degree angle.
7. Relocate the vein and decrease the needle angle slightly.
8. Slowly, with a downward motion followed immediately by a raising of the point, pick up the vein, leveling needle until it is almost flush with the skin.
9. On entering the vein there may be a backflow of blood which will indicate successful entry. There may be no blood return if the vein is small. Usually pinching the rubber tube just above the needle adapter and then releasing it will back the blood into the plastic tubing. If doubtful of the needle's position in the vein, check by this method. With experience the fingers will become sensitive to the needle's entering the vein—the resistance encountered as the needle meets the wall of the vein and the snap felt at the loss of resistance as the needle enters the lumen. This is more difficult to discern on thin-walled veins with small blood volume. To prevent a through puncture, move the needle slowly, checking at each movement for a backflow of blood.
10. Once the vein is entered, the needle is moved cautiously up the lumen for about three quarters of an inch.
11. Release the tourniquet.
12. Release the pressure exerted by the little finger, unkinking the tube and allowing the solution to flow.
13. Check carefully for any signs of swelling.

If the vein has sustained a through puncture (evidenced by a developing hematoma) and the venipuncture is unsuccessful, the needle should be immediately removed and pressure applied to the site. Never reapply a tourniquet to the extremity immediately after a venipuncture; a hematoma will occur, limiting veins and providing an excellent culture medium for bacteria.

ANCHORING NEEDLE AND SECURING ARMBOARD

To anchor the needle, carry out the following steps (see Figure 15):

1. Use 1 inch wide tape over the hub and shaft of the needle. Tape the needle flush with the skin—no elevation of the hub is necessary and it would only increase the risk of a through puncture from the point of the needle.
2. Place a one half inch strip of tape—adhesive up—under the hub of the needle. Place one end tightly and diagonally over the needle. Repeat with the other end, crossing over the first. This secures the needle firmly and prevents any sideward movement.
3. Loop the tubing and secure it with tape independently of the needle. This eliminates dislodging the needle by an accidental pull on the tubing.
4. Indicate the size of the needle and the date on the tape.

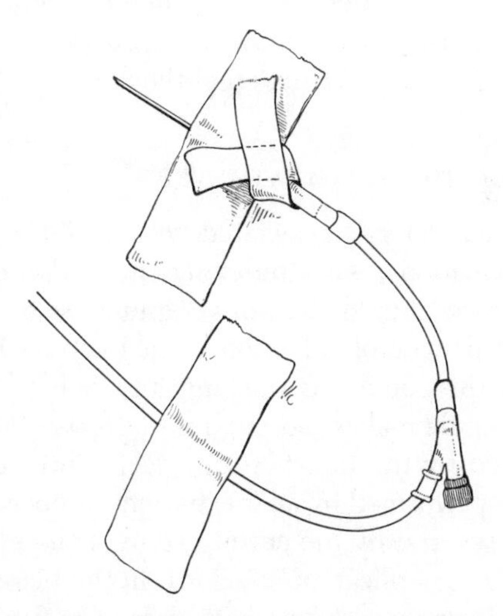

FIG. 15. Note that tape, securing tubing, is independent of needle; an accidental pull will not dislodge the needle.

This will help ensure removal of the needle within a safe period of time.

ARMBOARD. The use of an armboard is helpful in immobilizing the extremity when undue motion could result in an infiltration or a phlebitis. It is a valuable aid in restraining the arm when infusions are initiated on uncooperative, disoriented, or elderly patients or children, or when the needle is inserted on the dorsum of the hand or in an area of joint flexion. When the metacarpal veins are used the fingers should be immobilized to prevent any movement of the needle that could result in a phlebitis.

If a plastic armboard is used, cover it with absorbent paper or bandage to prevent the arm from perspiring and sticking to the board. Make certain that any tape placed on the needle is independent of the board so that a motion of the arm on the board will not cause a pull on the needle. If restraint of the arm is necessary, the restraint is secured to the board, not to the patient's arm above the puncture area; such restraint might act as a tourniquet, causing a backflow of blood into the needle, resulting in clotting and obstruction of the flow.

INSERTION OF THE INTRACATHETER

As the intracatheter is associated with a higher incidence of serious complications, only the experienced therapist, alert to the risks involved, should attempt venipuncture by this method. The inherent danger of infection from bacteria invading the vein through the cutaneous opening and being carried along the plastic cannula makes thorough skin preparation necessary. Trauma caused by the insertion of a large intracatheter is increased when performed by an inexperienced operator.

A catheter severed by the cutting edge of the needle can result in a serious complication when lost in the blood stream. An intracatheter introduced into a vein over joint flexion increases the risk of complication if the extremity is not immobilized.

A catheter facilitates prolonged therapy but increases the

risk of thrombophlebitis. A limited time before removal of the intracatheter reduces the incidence of phlebitis; a time limit is sometimes difficult to enforce, however, since veins may be exhausted in critically ill patients whose life depends upon infusion therapy.

To minimize the danger of infection, the Massachusetts General Hospital has devised "venipuncture sets" for insertion of all inlying plastic intravenous catheters. These sterile kits contain a disposable plastic razor, iodine, alcohol, a drape, disposable gloves, and Neosporin ointment. Moran et al. [5] performed studies that offer conclusive evidence that an antibiotic ointment containing neomycin, bacitracin, and polymyxin, applied daily to the puncture site, reduces the incidence of secondary infection.

Local anesthesia is often employed to prevent discomfort when a large catheter is used; more nerve endings are traumatized by the large catheter than by a small needle. Since the subcutaneous tissue is comparatively insensitive, most of the pain occurs as the needle penetrates the skin [2]. Usually 0.5 or 1 percent procaine is used. Because of a possible sensitivity to procaine the patient should be questioned as to allergies. A minimum amount of procaine is injected intradermally with a 25-gauge hypodermic needle to raise a wheal through which the intravenous needle is passed. Care must be observed to prevent an inadvertent intravascular injection.

Technique for Venipuncture and Installation of Plastic Needle

Steps to follow in placing a catheter mounted on a metal needle are as follows:

1. Apply tourniquet and select vein.
2. Shave the skin if necessary and prepare with iodine and alcohol or an accepted antiseptic.
3. Inject a local anesthetic intradermally if required.
4. Perform the venipuncture in the usual manner. When the needle has punctured the venous wall, introduce the needle one

half inch farther to ensure entry of the catheter into the lumen of the vein.

5. Hold the needle in place and slowly slide catheter hub until desired length is in the vein (see Figure 16). If the venipuncture is unsuccessful *do not reinsert the needle into the catheter;* to do so could sever the catheter.

6. Remove the needle by holding catheter hub in place. To minimize leakage of blood while removing the needle and connecting the infusion set, apply pressure on the vein beyond the catheter with the little finger (see Figure 17).

7. Attach the administration set which has been previously cleared of air and regulate the rate of flow.

8. Apply Neosporin ointment.

9. Tape catheter securely to prevent any motion which could contribute to phlebitis. Avoid taping over the injection site if antibiotic ointment is to be applied daily. Cover injection site with a sterile sponge.

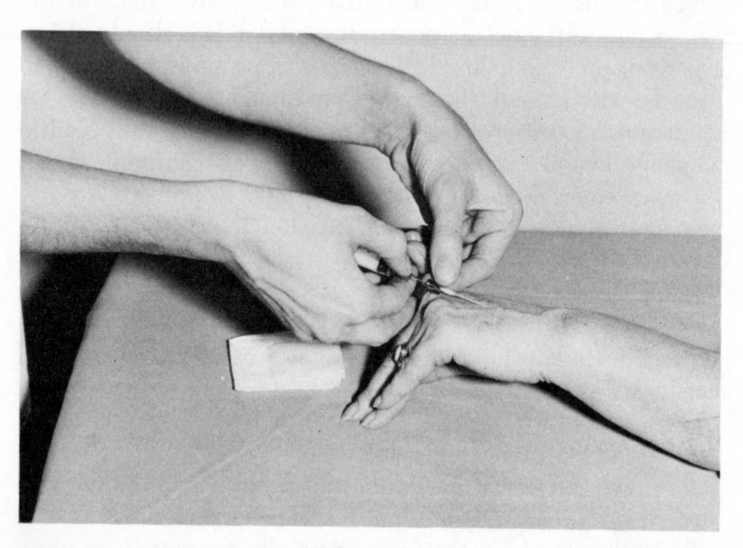

FIG. 16. Hub of the needle is held in place while catheter (Jelco I.V.) is slipped off the shaft until desired length is in the vein. (Jelco Laboratories, Raritan, N.J.)

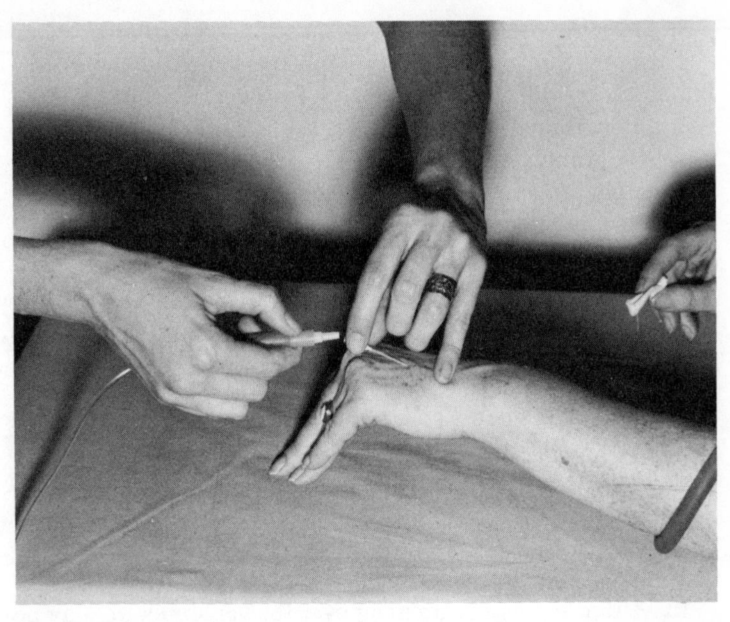

FIG. 17. Pressure on vein reduces leakage of blood which occurs when the needle is withdrawn from the catheter (Jelco I.V.) and the catheter is connected to the infusion set. (Jelco Laboratories, Raritan, N.J.)

10. Loop tubing and tape independent of the catheter to prevent an accidental pull from withdrawing the catheter.
11. Indicate date of insertion and size and type of the catheter on the tape.

CATHETER INSERTED THROUGH THE NEEDLE

Although certain precautions must be observed, the same principles just listed are employed when the longer catheter is threaded through the needle.

1. Apply tourniquet and select vein.
2. Shave the skin if necessary and apply an accepted antiseptic.

3. Make the venipuncture.
4. Gently thread catheter through the lumen of the needle into the vein until the desired length has been introduced.
5. Apply digital pressure on the vein to hold the catheter in place; withdraw the needle.
6. Apply pressure with a sterile sponge for 30 seconds to minimize bleeding through the puncture site.
7. Attach the needle to the infusion set and regulate the rate.
8. Slip the shield from the base of the needle over the bevel and tape; the shield must be kept in place to protect the cutting edge of the needle and prevent severing the catheter. A tongue depressor is frequently used to secure the needle and catheter to further guard against kinking and breaking of the catheter at the junction of the needle.
9. Tape the catheter to prevent motion.
10. Indicate date of insertion and type and size of catheter on tape.
11. Apply Neosporin ointment.
12. A sterile pressure dressing over the venipuncture may be required for a short time; the puncture made by the needle is larger than the inlying catheter and seepage of fluid may occur.
13. An armboard should be used if the catheter lies over a point of flexion—motion contributes to phlebitis. The arm must not be fastened tightly to the armboard; vascular occlusion results in a plugged catheter and stasis edema may occur.

If the venipuncture is unsuccessful the needle and catheter must be removed *together;* to pull the catheter through the needle may sever the catheter and result in its loss in the circulation.

Intravenous catheterization by surgical procedure

When lack of superficial veins prevents venipuncture, a surgical procedure for exposure and cannulation of the vein is performed by the physician. The commonest technique is insertion of the cannula or catheter into the exposed vein through the incision. This makes skin approximation difficult and may lead to a delay in healing and an increased risk of bacterial invasion in the vein through the incision.

Dudley [3] describes a modified technique in which the incision is made in the usual manner to expose the vein. The cannula is then inserted slightly distal to the incision through a nick in the skin made by a small scalpel knife. The cannula is then introduced into the exposed vein in the usual manner. Later removal of the cannula does not disturb the incision.

REFERENCES

1. Abbott Laboratories. *Parenteral Administration.* North Chicago, Ill., 1969. P. 10.
2. Adriani, J. Venipuncture. *American Journal of Nursing* 62:66, 1962.
3. Dudley, H. A. F. Modified technique for intravenous cannulation. *Surgery, Gynecology & Obstetrics* 111:513, 1960.
4. Metheny, N. M., and Sniveley, W. D., Jr. *Nurses' Handbook of Fluid Balance.* Philadelphia: Lippincott, 1967. Pp. 147, 110–115.
5. Moran, J. M., Atwood, R. P., and Rowe, M. I. A clinical and bacteriologic study of infections associated with venous cutdown. *New England Journal of Medicine* 272:554, 1965.
6. Pfizer Laboratories. Intravenous techniques. *Spectrum* 9:2–5, 1965.
7. Welt, L. *Clinical Disorders of Hydration and Acid-Base Equilibrium* (2d ed.). Boston: Little, Brown, 1959. P. 131.

5.
The Staff Nurse's Responsibility in Maintenance of Infusions

SAFE, SUCCESSFUL, FLUID THERAPY depends not only upon the knowledge and skill of the intravenous nurse, but also upon the role the staff nurse plays in maintaining the infusion. The proper rate must be maintained, medications must be infused at their allotted time, and potential hazards prevented.

STERILE TECHNIQUE

There is a great risk of infection if sterile technique is not observed. Solutions, once opened, must be used within 24 hours or discarded. Glucose is a culture medium and when exposed to air for an extended length of time becomes a potential vehicle for bacteria.

Prolonged intravenous therapy presents a hazard. To minimize the risk of a deep phlebitis during a constant infusion, the tubing should be changed every 24 hours, using rigid sterile technique and making sure all air is expelled from the tubing before attaching to the inlying needle.

AMBULATING PATIENTS WITH INFUSIONS

Special precautions must be taken when ambulating patients with infusions. The fluid flask must be kept sufficiently high at all times to maintain a constant flow. Any cessation in the rate must be detected immediately and remedied before a clot is allowed to plug the needle.

Fluid maintenance requires frequent observation of patients receiving infusions. The attending nurse should visit the patient every hour, checking the rate of flow, the amount of solution remaining, and the site of infusion, as described in the following sections.

Rate of flow

Since the rate of flow, once established, is often difficult to maintain, the staff nurse should check and readjust the flow whenever necessary. When an infusion stops, the cause must be immediately investigated and remedied.

When infusion stops

The following procedure is to be used when the infusion stops:

1. Check for infiltration.
2. Check the fluid level in the bottle.
3. Check for kinking of the tubing.
4. Open the clamp.
5. Check air vent (has it been inserted if required and is it patent?).
6. Check the needle for patency by kinking the tubing a few inches from the needle while pinching and releasing the tubing between the needle and the kinked tubing. Resistence if encountered should be treated with caution as a clot may have plugged the needle. If a patient complains of pain, a sclerosed vein may be the cause of the cessation of flow. In either case the needle must be removed.
7. Is the needle in line with the vein or up against the wall of the vein? A slight adjustment, by moving the needle, may remedy the problem.
8. If the solution is cold, as in the case of blood, venous spasm may result. Heat placed directly on the vein will

relieve the spasm and increase the flow of the infusion.

9. If the infusion is blood, check the filter; heavy sediment may be slowing the flow. Replace the filter if necessary.
10. Increase the height of the bottle to increase gravity.
11. If unable to restart the infusion after these procedures have been followed, the intravenous must be restarted.

AMOUNT OF SOLUTION IN FLASKS

Air and *blood embolism* are significant hazards of infusion therapy and may be associated with delay in changing solution bottles. A fresh bottle of solution should be added before the level of fluid falls in the drip chamber. Failure to do this results in the following problems:

1. *Plugged needle.* Intravenous solutions flow into the vein by means of gravity. Once the fluid level has dropped in the tubing to about the level of the patient's chest, the blood will be forced back into the needle causing a clot to form. This clot could prove fatal to the patient if positive pressure is applied in an attempt to flush the needle.
2. *Trapped air.* If the bottle is changed after the level of fluid drops in the tubing and before the needle plugs, the air is trapped in the tubing and forced into the patient by pressure of the fresh solution. A fatal air embolism can result. According to Mollison [2], when a blood container is allowed to run empty, and there is a negative pressure in the vein being used for the infusion, air may be drawn into the blood stream. He states, "It is easy to introduce air into the patient's veins at the beginning or when changing from one bottle to another." Infusions through a central venous catheter carry an even greater risk of air embolism than those infused through a peripheral vein. Since the central venous pressure is lower than the peripheral pressure there is a greater chance of a negative pressure causing air to be sucked into the patient's circulation when the bottle runs dry. According to

Metheny and Snively [1], "Small amounts of air are not always harmful, yet as little as 10 ml may be fatal in some patients."

Before the flow ceases and the bottle empties, replace the empty bottle with fresh solution using the following procedure:

1. Vent fresh bottle if vent is required.
2. Kink tubing to prevent air from being introduced into the flowing solution.
3. Change flask. Hang solution bottle before unkinking tubing.
4. Readjust rate if necessary.

Infiltration or inflammation at injection site

Failure to recognize an infiltration before the swelling has increased to a sizable degree may:

1. Cause damage to the tissues.
2. Prevent the patient from receiving necessary and urgent medication.
3. Limit available veins for future therapy.

If the question of infiltration exists, compare the questionable extremity with the normal extremity. An intravenous has infiltrated if

1. There is swelling about the site of the needle.
2. A tourniquet applied above the needle does not stop the flow of fluid.

Checking for an infiltration by a backflow of blood into the adapter is not a reliable method for the following reasons:

1. In small veins the needle may approach the size of the vein, occluding the lumen and obstructing the flow of

blood; the solution flows undiluted so that no back flow of blood is obtained.

2. The needle may have punctured the vein causing an infiltration and at the same time be within the lumen of the vein, or the bevel may be only partially within the lumen of the vein, causing a swelling and still producing a backflow of blood on test.

Infiltration or inflammation require removal of the infusion.

Termination of infusion

To terminate the infusion follow this procedure:

1. Stop flow by clamping off tubing.
2. Remove all tape from needle.
3. With a dry sterile sponge held over the injection site, remove needle. The needle must be removed nearly flush with the skin. This prevents the point from damaging the posterior wall of the vein, thus encouraging the process of thrombosis.
4. Apply pressure instantly and firmly. Do not rub. Hematomas occur from needles carelessly removed and render veins useless for future use.

BAND-AID. Band-Aids should not be used unless specifically ordered. It must be emphasized that a Band-Aid is not used to stop bleeding and does not take the place of pressure. If ordered, it should be applied only after pressure has been applied and the bleeding stopped.

REFERENCES

1. Metheny, N. M., and Snively, W. D., Jr. *Nurses' Handbook of Fluid Balance*. Philadelphia: Lippincott, 1967. P. 138.
2. Mollison, P. L. *Blood Transfusion in Clinical Medicine* (3d ed.). Springfield, Ill.: Thomas, 1961. Pp. 574–575.

6.

Rate of Administration of Parenteral Infusions

One of the prime considerations in the administration of parenteral solutions is the rate of flow. Ideally the physician orders the rate of flow since in determining the rate he must consider the solution, the patient's condition, and the effect he wishes to produce. The nurse who initiates the infusion or who cares for its maintenance is responsible for regulating and maintaining the proper rate of administration. Occasionally when the rate has not been ordered the nurse must assume this responsibility.

DETERMINING FACTORS FOR INFUSION RATE

To determine the flow rate intelligently, the nurse must have a knowledge of parenteral solutions, their effect, and rate of administration. She must also understand other factors that influence the speed of the infusion. These factors include (1) surface area of the body, (2) condition of the patient, (3) age of the patient, (4) composition of the fluid, and (5) the patient's tolerance to the infusion.

SURFACE AREA OF THE BODY. The body surface area is proportionate to many essential physiological processes (organ size, blood volume, respiration, and heat loss) and therefore to the total metabolic activity. It provides a helpful guide for determining fluids and electrolytes and for computing rate of infusions. The larger an individual, the more fluid and nutrients he requires and the faster he can utilize them. The usual infusion rate is 3 ml per square meter of body surface per minute (see Nomograms for determining surface area, Chapter 9, Figure 23). This rate applies to maintenance and replacement fluids [5]. However, the speed must be carefully adjusted to each individual.

CONDITION OF PATIENT. Since the heart and the kidneys play a vital role in the utilization of infused solutions, the cardiac and renal status of the patient affects the desired rate of administration. An expanded blood volume may occur when fluids, rapidly infused, overtax an impaired heart and renal damage causes retention of fluid. Patients suffering from hypovolemia must receive plasma and blood rapidly, but the desired speed of the infusion may be affected by impairment of the homeostatic controls. Therefore the rate should be specified by the physician. Vital signs must be carefully observed and the speed of the infusion decreased as the blood pressure rises.

AGE OF PATIENT. Because there is usually some degree of cardiac and renal damage in the elderly, fluids are administered slowly to prevent an increase in venous pressure which could result in pulmonary edema and cardiovascular disturbances [5]. Infants and small children are particularly prone to pulmonary edema when excessive quantities of fluid or rapidly infused fluids expand the vascular system [5]. The rate of administration must be determined by the physician and all precautions observed to ensure steady maintenance at the required rate of flow. If difficulty is encountered in controlling a constant rate, it should be reported and corrected at once.

The special pediatric infusion sets which deliver a smaller size drop (50 to 60 drops per milliliter) provide precision control of the rate of flow. The infusion pumps, such as the Holter pump* are valuable in maintaining the exact rate of flow regardless of difficulties.

COMPOSITION OF FLUID. The composition of fluid affects the rate of flow. When the solution is used as a vehicle for administering drugs, the speed of the infusion depends upon the drug and the effect the physician wishes to produce. Potassium, because of its deleterious effect on the heart when infused at a rapid rate should be administered with caution. "About 40 mEq. of potassium over an eight-hour period is an average rate for administering potassium parenterally. In emergencies, the rate of administration may be up to four times as fast" [4].

Concentration of solutions must be considered since the flow rate may alter the desired effect. When dextrose is administered for caloric benefits it is infused at a rate that will ensure complete utilization. Dextrose can be administered at a maximum speed of 0.5 gm per kilogram per hour [5, 7] without producing glycosuria in a normal individual. At this rate it would take approximately 1½ hours to administer a liter of 5 percent dextrose to an individual weighing 70 kg or twice as long for a liter of 10 percent dextrose [7]. This maximum rate is faster than usual and not customarily used except in an emergency.

When a diuretic effect is desired a more rapid infusion is necessary. If the solution is too rapidly infused for complete metabolism, the glucose accumulates in the blood stream, increases the osmolality, and acts as a diuretic.

When oliguria or anuria occurs, the status of the kidneys must be determined before solutions containing potassium can be administered. Urinary suppression may be due to a blood volume deficit or to kidney damage. An initial hydrating solution, to test kidney function, is usually administered at a rate of 8 ml per square meter of body surface per minute for 45 minutes [2]. If urinary flow is not accomplished the rate is slowed to about 2 ml per square meter of body surface per

* Extracorporeal Medical Specialities, Inc., Mt. Laurel, N.J.

minute for another hour. If urinary output has not occurred after this period, it is presumed kidney damage is present [2, 5].

TOLERANCE. Tolerance to solutions varies with individuals and influences the rate of infusion. A 5 percent solution of alcohol can be administered at the rate of 200 to 300 ml per hour to sedate without intoxication in the average adult [5]. However, the rate must be adjusted to the individual.

When protein hydrolysates are infused, a slower rate of administration, 2 ml per minute, is necessary to test the patient's sensitivity to the protein [7]. Nausea and a feeling of warmth may occur from excessively rapid administration; if these symptoms do not subside when the rate of administration is decreased, the infusion should be stopped [5].

COMPUTATION OF RATE OF FLOW

Frequently the doctor orders a total volume of fluid to be infused over a 24-hour period. If the nurse knows the volume and the flow rate of the administration set in use, she can easily compute the required rate of flow. A quick, easy formula for computing flow rate in drops (gtt) per minute is

$$\frac{\text{gtt/ml of given set}}{\text{60 (min in hour)}} \times \text{total hourly volume} = \text{gtt/min}$$

If a set delivers 15 drops per milliliter and 240 ml are to be infused in 1 hour,

$$\frac{15}{60} \times 240 = \frac{1}{4} \times 240 = 60 \text{ gtt/min}$$

Whenever a 15 drops per milliliter set is used, merely divide the hourly volume to be infused by 4 and the number of drops a minute will be obtained.

If the set delivers 10 drops per milliliter, divide the number of milliliters to be infused by 6 for drops per minute:

$$\frac{10}{60} \times \text{hourly volume} = \frac{1}{6} \times \text{hourly volume} = \text{gtt/min}$$

Manufacturers of parenteral solutions have devised convenient calculators to assist the nurse in accurate rate determinations (see Figure 18). The Normosol Calculator by Abbott

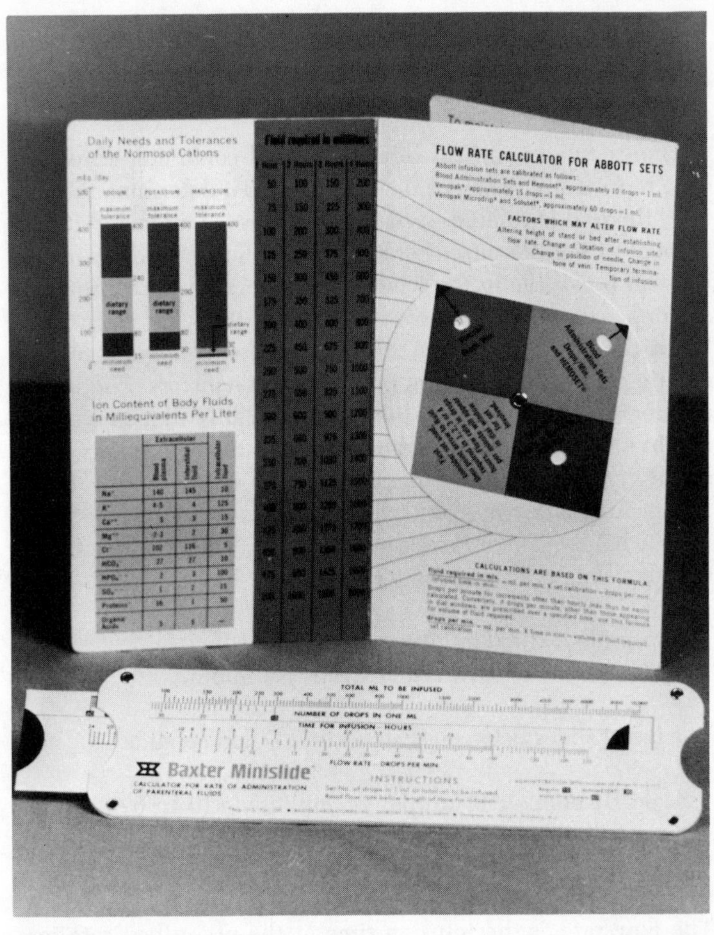

FIG. 18. Handy calculators for determining rate of flow of a given volume of fluid over a set period of time. (Normosol Calculator, Abbott Laboratories, North Chicago, Ill.; Minislide, Travenol Laboratories, Morton Grove, Ill.)

Laboratories is a concise, excellent device for calculating both rate determinations and surface area in square meters. The rate determinator is devised for use with Abbott sets or sets calculated as follows:

Fluid administration sets approximately	15 gtt = 1 ml
Blood administration sets approximately	10 gtt = 1 ml
Pediatric administration sets approximately	60 gtt = 1 ml

The calculator consists of a rotary dial containing three sectors, representing each of the three sets. To determine the flow rate, the dial is rotated until the set in use is aligned with the amount of fluid required for 1, 2, 3, or 4 hours. Drops per minute will be visible in the window contained in the represented sector.

On the opposite side a dial provides a nomogram for calculating surface area of the body in square meters. The weight in kilograms or pounds on the rotary wheel is aligned with the height in centimeters or inches. An indicator then points to the surface area in square meters.

The Minislide by Baxter Laboratories provides the nurse with a handy, quick device for computing fluid rates. It consists of a slide rule containing four scales:

Top, scale A: total milliliters to be infused
Bottom, scale D: flow rate in drops per minute

The insert slides between scales A and D and contains

Scale B: number of drops per milliliter (10 to 60) a given set delivers
Scale C: time in hours for infusion

The flow rate or the infusion time at the prescribed rate may be determined by sliding the insert until the number of drops that the set delivers is aligned with total milliliters to be infused. Opposite the time (hours) for infusion, see drops required per minute; opposite the prescribed flow rate, see the infusion time (hours).

FACTORS AFFECTING THE FLOW RATE

The infusion should be checked frequently to maintain the required rate of flow. Due to certain factors, the rate is subject to change.

HEIGHT OF THE SOLUTION BOTTLE. Intravenous fluids run by gravity. Any change in gravity by raising or lowering the infusion bottle will change the rate of flow. When patients receiving infusions are ambulated or transported to x-ray, the solution bottle should be retained at the same height, or the speed of the infusion readjusted to maintain the prescribed rate of flow.

CLOT IN THE NEEDLE. Any temporary stoppage of the infusion, such as a delay in changing infusion bottles, may cause a clot to form in the lumen of the needle, partially or completely obstructing it. Clot formation may also occur when an increase in venous pressure in the infusion arm forces blood back into the needle. This results from restriction of the venous circulation and is most commonly caused by (1) the blood pressure cuff on the infusion arm, (2) restraints placed on or above the infusion needle, and (3) the patient's lying on the arm receiving the intravenous [3].

CHANGE IN POSITION OF THE NEEDLE. A change in the needle's position may push the bevel of the needle against or away from the wall of the vein [6]. Special precautions should be taken to prevent speed shock or overloading the vascular system by making sure the solution is flowing freely before adjusting the rate.

CHANGE IN TEMPERATURE OR COMPOSITION OF THE SOLUTION. Stimulation of the vasoconstrictors from any infusion of cold blood or irritating solution may cause venous spasm, impeding the rate of flow [6]. A warm pack placed on the vein proximal to the infusion needle will offset this reaction.

TRAUMA TO THE VEIN. Any injury such as phlebitis or thrombosis which reduces the lumen of the vein will decrease the flow of the solution.

PLUGGED VENT. A plugged vent in the solution bottle will cause the infusion to stop [1]. Check the vent needle for patency.

If there is any question as to the rate of administration, the therapist should check with the physician. This applies to intravenous administration of drugs in solution. The rates should also be established on patients receiving two or more infusions simultaneously. Any change in the rate from that normally used should be ordered by the attending physician.

The nurse should never exert positive pressure (manual pressure) to infuse solutions or blood. This should be the responsibility of the physician.

REFERENCES

1. Abbott Laboratories. *Parenteral Administration.* North Chicago, Ill., 1969. P. 19.
2. Abbott Laboratories. *Fluid and Electrolytes.* North Chicago, Ill., 1960. P. 32.
3. Bard, C. R., Inc. *An Outline for the Use of IV Placement Units.* Murray Hill, N.J., 1970. P. 8.
4. Crowell, C. E., and Staff of Educational Design, Inc., N.Y. Potassium imbalance. *American Journal of Nursing* 67:358, 1967.
5. Metheny, N. M., and Snively, W. D., Jr. *Nurses' Handbook of Fluid Balance.* Philadelphia: Lippincott, 1967. Pp. 118–124, 256.
6. Pfizer Laboratories. Intravenous techniques. *Spectrum* 9:2, 1965.
7. Williams, J. T., and Moravec, D. F. *Intravenous Therapy.* Hammond, Ind.: Clissold Publishing, 1967. P. 49.

7. Hazards and Complications of Intravenous Therapy

INTRAVENOUS THERAPY subjects the patient to numerous hazards, many of which can be avoided if the nurse understands the risks involved and uses all available measures to prevent their occurrence. The *local complications* occur most frequently and include thrombophlebitis and infiltrations. The *systemic complications* are the most serious and consist of the following:

1. Pyrogenic reactions
2. Pulmonary embolism resulting from
   a) Blood emboli—"clots"
   b) Air emboli—"bubbles"
3. Pulmonary edema
4. Speed shock

LOCAL COMPLICATIONS

Occasionally local complications are not recognized until considerable damage is done. Early recognition may prevent (1) extensive edema depriving the patient of urgently needed fluid and medications, (2) necrosis, and (3) thrombophlebitis with the subsequent danger of embolism. The local complications occur as the result of trauma to the wall of the vein.

Thrombus

Any injury that roughens the endothelial cells of the venous wall allows platelets to adhere and a thrombus to form. Because the point of the needle traumatizes the wall of the vein where it touches, thrombi form on the vein and at the tip of the needle [11]. It must be remembered that thrombi form an excellent trap for bacteria, whether carried by the blood stream from an infection in a remote part of the body or introduced through the subcutaneous orifice [3].

Thrombophlebitis

Thrombophlebitis is the term used to denote a twofold injury: thrombus plus inflammation. The development of thrombophlebitis is easily recognized. A painful inflammation develops along the length of the vein. If the infusion is allowed to continue, the vein progressively thromboses, becoming hard, tortuous, tender, and painful [7]. Early detection may prevent an obstructive thrombophlebitis which causes the infusion to slow and finally stop. This condition is most painful, persisting indefinitely, incapacitating the patient, and limiting valuable veins for future therapy.

Usually a sterile inflammation develops from a chemical or mechanical irritation. When the inflammation is the result of sepsis it is much more serious and carries with it the potential danger of septicemia and acute bacterial endocarditis.

There is always the inherent danger of embolism when a thrombosis occurs. The more pronounced the inflammation and the more intense the pain, the more organized the thrombus is apt to become. It has been frequently stated that an embolism is less likely to occur from the well-attached clot of thrombophlebitis than from phlebothrombosis [6].

Phlebothrombosis

Phlebothrombosis denotes thrombosis and is a pertinent term usually indicating that the inflammation is relatively inconspicuous. It is thought to give rise to embolism since the thrombus is poorly attached to the wall of the vein [6]. Both processes have a degree of inflammation and are associated with potential embolism.

CONTRIBUTING FACTORS. Any irritation involving the wall of the vein predisposes the patient to thrombophlebitis. Inflammation to the vein will occur from any foreign body under certain conditions: (1) duration of the infusion, (2) composition of the solution, (3) site of the infusion, (4) technique, and (5) method employed [2].

Duration of the infusion is a significant factor in the development of thrombophlebitis. As the duration of time is lengthened, the incidence and degree of inflammation increase. Infusions left in place over 24 hours are prime offenders [2, 4].

The *composition of the solution* may play a role. Venous irritation and inflammation may result from the infusion of hypertonic glucose solutions, certain drug additives, or from solutions with a pH significantly different from that of the plasma. Solutions of dextrose are known to be irritating to the vein [4, 5]. The USP specifications for pH of dextrose solutions range from 3.5 to 6.5; acidity is necessary to prevent caramelization of the dextrose during autoclaving and to preserve the stability of the solution during storage. Studies have been performed which show a significant reduction in thrombophlebitis when buffered glucose solutions have been infused [5]. Abbott Manufacturing Company, recognizing this problem, identifies the pH of each solution and provides Neut, a sodium bicarbonate 1 percent additive solution, to increase the pH of acid intravenous solutions. This additive, however, poses a problem of incompatibility when added to solutions containing drugs. Abbott's circular on Neut calls attention to the precaution that "When Neut is added to solutions, the compatibility of these solutions with other drugs may be altered." According to Williams [14], "It is quite likely that changes in pH produce the largest number of incompatibilities." As an example tetracycline hydrochloride, with a pH of from 2.5 to 3.0, is unstable in an alkaline environment.

The *site of infusion* can be a factor contributing to thrombophlebitis. The veins in areas over joint flexion undergo injury when motion of the needle irritates the venous wall. The veins in the lower extremities are especially prone to trauma, enhanced by the stagnant blood in varicosities and the stasis in the peripheral venous circulation.

Small veins are subject to inflammation when used to infuse an irritating solution; the infusion needle may occlude the entire lumen of the vein, obstructing the flow of circulating blood; the solution then flows undiluted, irritating the wall of the vein.

Technique can mean the difference between a successful infusion and the complication of thrombophlebitis. Only minimum trauma results from a venipuncture skillfully executed, whereas a carelessly performed venipuncture may seriously traumatize the venous wall.

Phlebitis associated with sepsis may be related to the technique of the operator. There is always the risk of infection if sterile technique is not zealously observed. Thorough cleansing of the skin is important in preventing infections. Maintenance of asepsis is essential during long-term therapy, particularly in the use of the intracatheter [10].

Methods employed to infuse parenteral solutions may foster a septic thrombophlebitis. This complication is most often associated with the intracatheter. The intracatheter threaded through the needle remains sterile, does not come in contact with the skin, but provides a large subcutaneous orifice facilitating entry of bacteria around the catheter and seepage of fluid.

The catheter mounted on the needle is not without fault as it comes in direct contact with the skin before being introduced into the vein. However, the tight fit through the skin may bar further bacterial entry.

PREVENTIVE MEASURES. In performing venipunctures, the therapist should exercise every caution to avoid injuring the wall of the vein needlessly. Multiple punctures, through-and-through punctures, and damage to the posterior wall of the vein with the point of the needle can cause thrombosis. The risk of phlebitis may be minimized if the nurse

1. Refrains from using veins in the lower extremities
2. Selects veins with ample blood volume when infusing irritating substances
3. Avoids veins in areas over joint flexion
4. Anchors needles securely to prevent motion

To prevent a septic phlebitis, thorough preparation of the skin, together with aseptic technique and maintenance of asepsis during infusion, is imperative.

Periodic inspection of the injection site will detect developing complications before serious damage occurs. Complaints of a painful infusion make it necessary to differentiate between an early phlebitis and venospasm from an irritating solution. If the latter, slowing the solution and applying heat to the vein will dilate the vessel and increase the blood flow, diluting the solution and relieving the pain. Following hypertonic solutions with isotonic fluids will flush the vein of irritating substances.

If inflammation accompanies the pain, a change in the injection site should be considered. To continue the infusion will only bring progressive trauma and limit available veins. An enforced time limit for removal of the needle reduces the incidence of phlebitis [2, 4].

When removing the infusion needle, care must be taken to prevent injury to the wall of the vein; the needle should be removed at an angle nearly flush with the skin. Pressure should be applied for a reasonable length of time to prevent extravasation of blood.

Infiltration

Dislodgment of the needle with consequent infiltration of fluid is not uncommon and is too frequently considered of

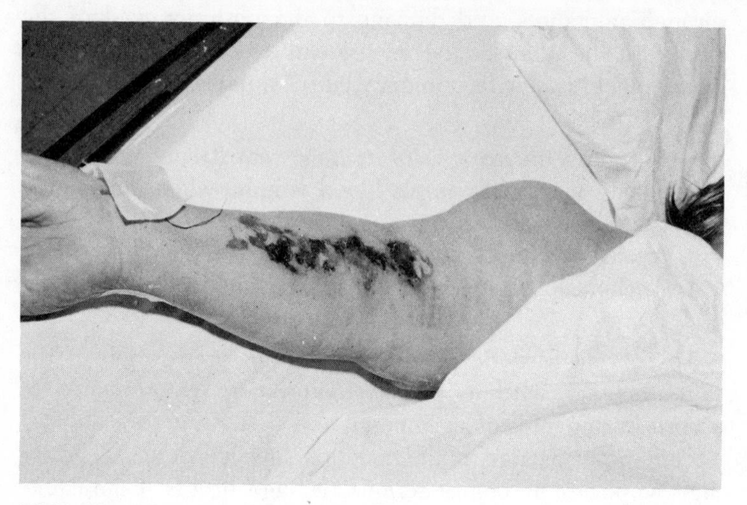

FIG. 19. Necrosis of tissues resulting from infiltration of concentrated solution of potassium chloride.

minor significance. With the increasing numbers of irritating solutions and the frequency with which potent drugs are infused via intravenous solutions, serious problems may occur when the fluid invades the surrounding tissues. Hypertonic, acid, and alkaline solutions are contraindicated for hypodermoclysis and not intended for other than venous infusions. If allowed to infiltrate, necrosis could occur (see Figures 19 and 20).

If necrosis is avoided, edema may nevertheless

1. Deprive the patient of fluid and drug absorption at the rate essential for successful therapy
2. Limit available veins for venipuncture, complicating therapy
3. Predispose the patient to infection

Extravasation can easily be recognized by the increasing edema at the site of the infusion. A comparison of the infusion

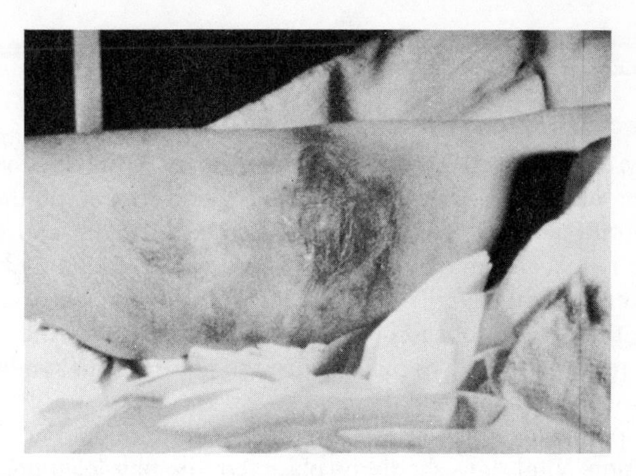

FIG. 20. Necrosis from hypertonic solution.

area with the identical area in the opposite extremity assists in determining whether there is a swelling.

Frequently the edema is allowed to increase to great proportions because of a misconception that a backflow of blood into the adapter is significant proof that the infusion is entering the vein. This is not a reliable method for checking a possible infiltration. The point of the needle may puncture the posterior wall of the vein, leaving the greater portion of the bevel within the lumen of the vein. Blood return will be obtained on negative pressure, but if the infusion is allowed to continue fluid will seep into the tissues at the point of the needle, increasing the edema.

Occasionally a blood return is not obtained on negative pressure. This may occur when the needle occludes the lumen of a small vein, obstructing the flow of blood.

To confirm an infiltration, apply a tourniquet tightly enough to restrict the venous flow, proximal to the injection site. If regardless of this venous obstruction the infusion continues, extravasation is evident.

Once an infiltration has occurred the needle should be removed immediately.

SYSTEMIC COMPLICATIONS

Pyrogenic reactions

Pyrogenic reactions occur when pyrogens (proteins foreign to the blood) are introduced into the blood stream, producing a febrile reaction. This sudden occurrence of chills and fever may be accompanied by general malaise, headache and, depending on the severity of the reaction, backache, nausea, and vomiting. If the infusion is allowed to continue, the increased absorption of pyrogens may induce the more serious symptoms of vascular collapse and shock.

A pyrogenic reaction calls for immediate termination of the infusion. Vital signs should be observed, the physician notified, and the solution saved for any necessary cultures.

The improvement in equipment (disposable plastic infusion sets) and the use of commercially prepared solutions have greatly reduced the number of pyrogenic reactions. Still, reactions do occur. Special precautions can reduce the incidence of pyrogenic reactions.

USE OF PYROGEN-FREE SOLUTIONS. The solution should be carefully inspected for abnormal cloudiness or for the presence of extraneous particulate matter which may represent fungi.

Methods of sterilization of parenteral fluids vary with manufacturing companies. If the method used produces a vacuum in solution bottles, presence of a vacuum should be noted; lack of vacuum indicates possible loss of sterility and contamination.

USE OF FRESHLY OPENED SOLUTIONS. Protein solutions, such as albumin and protein hydrolysates, must be used as soon as the seal is broken. To refrigerate these opened solutions for future use can result in serious consequence.

Other solutions should be used within 24 hours. The wise practice of indicating on the bottle the time and date that the seal is broken safeguards patients from possible contaminated infusions, especially patients on "keep-open" infusions for intermittent drug therapy.

PROTECTION OF SOLUTION FROM CONTAMINATION. In the drug-additive program, sterile technique is essential to prevent organisms from being introduced into the solution. All drugs must be reconstituted with a sterile diluent. Once opened, any unused diluent should be discarded.

Keep-open solutions, terminated temporarily for blood infusion or drug therapy, must be protected from contamination. Sterile caps are available for some containers; sterile sponges may provide protection.

Pulmonary embolism

Pulmonary embolism occurs when a substance, usually a blood clot, becomes free floating and is propelled by the venous circulation to the right side of the heart and on into the pulmonary artery [6]. Emboli may obstruct the main pulmonary artery or the arteries to the lobes, occluding arterial apertures at major bifurcations [6]. Obstruction of the main artery results in circulatory and cardiac disturbances. Recurrent small emboli may eventually result in pulmonary hypertension and right heart failure [8].

PREVENTIVE MEASURES. Certain precautions must be taken to prevent this serious complication from occurring.

1. Blood or plasma must be infused through an adequate filter to remove any particulate matter which could result in small emboli.
2. Veins on the lower extremities should be avoided when venipunctures are performed. These veins are particularly prone to trauma, predisposing the patient to thrombophlebitis. Although superficial veins rarely seem to be the source of emboli of consequence [6], a thrombosis may extend into the deep veins resulting in a potentially viable clot; superficial and deep veins unite freely in the lower extremities.

3. Positive pressure should not be employed to relieve clot formation. To check for patency of the lumen of the needle, kink the infusion tubing about eight inches from the needle. Then kink and release the tubing between the needle and the pinched tubing—if the tubing becomes hard and meets with resistance, obstruction is evident, necessitating removal and reinstatement of the infusion.

4. Special precautions should be observed in the drug-additive program. Reconstituted drugs must be completely dissolved before being added to parenteral solutions; it is the inherent nature of red cells to adhere to particles, adding to the danger of clot formation.

5. Solutions should be examined to detect any particulate matter.

AIR EMBOLISM. Air embolism is a significant possible complication of every infusion, although its occurrence is usually associated with blood infused under pressure. A fatal embolism may occur when small bubbles accumulate dangerously and form tenacious bubbles that block the pulmonary capillaries [1]. Recognition of the circumstances which contribute to this hazard and measures taken to prevent their occurrence are imperative for safe fluid therapy.

Infusions run by gravity. If the container is allowed to run dry, air enters the tubing and the fluid level drops to the proximity of the patient's chest. The pressure exerted by the blood on the walls of the veins controls the level to which the air drops in the tubing. A negative pressure in the vein may allow air to enter the blood stream. A negative pressure occurs when the extremity receiving the infusion is elevated above the heart [9]. Infusions flowing through a central venous catheter carry an even greater risk of air emboli when the flask empties than those flowing through a peripheral vein; since the central venous pressure is less than the peripheral venous pressure, there is more apt to be a negative pressure which could suck air into the circulation.

If the fluid bottle on a continuous infusion should empty,

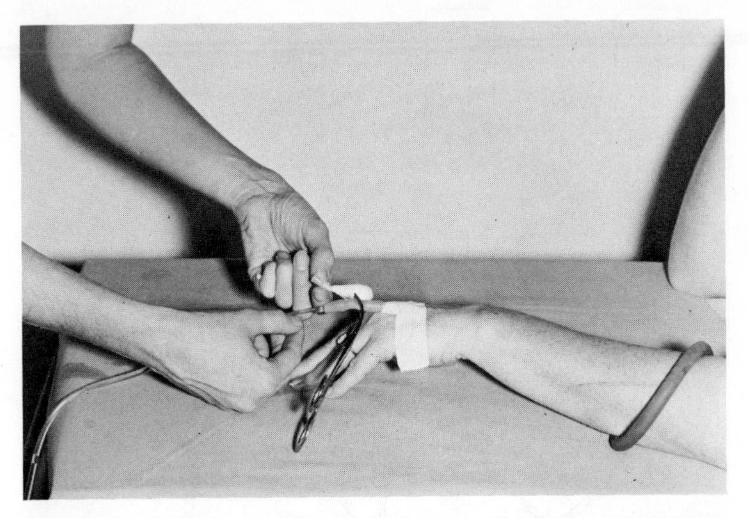

FIG. 21. Removing air from infusion set. The hemostat prevents air from entering the vein while a sterile needle allows air to escape from administration set.

fresh solution will force the trapped air into the circulation. To remove the air from the administration set (see Figure 21):

1. Place a hemostat close to the infusion needle.
2. Hang the fresh solution.
3. With an antiseptic, clean the rubber section of the tubing proximal to the hemostat and below the air level in the tubing.
4. Insert a sterile needle to allow the air to escape.
5. Remove clamp and readjust flow.

The Y-type infusion set (see Figure 22) is a less obvious source but one by which great quantities of air can be drawn into the blood stream. Running solutions simultaneously is the contributing factor. If one container empties, it becomes the source of air for the flowing solution. This is explained by the fact that the atmospheric pressure is greater in the open tubing to the empty bottle than below the partially restricted clamp

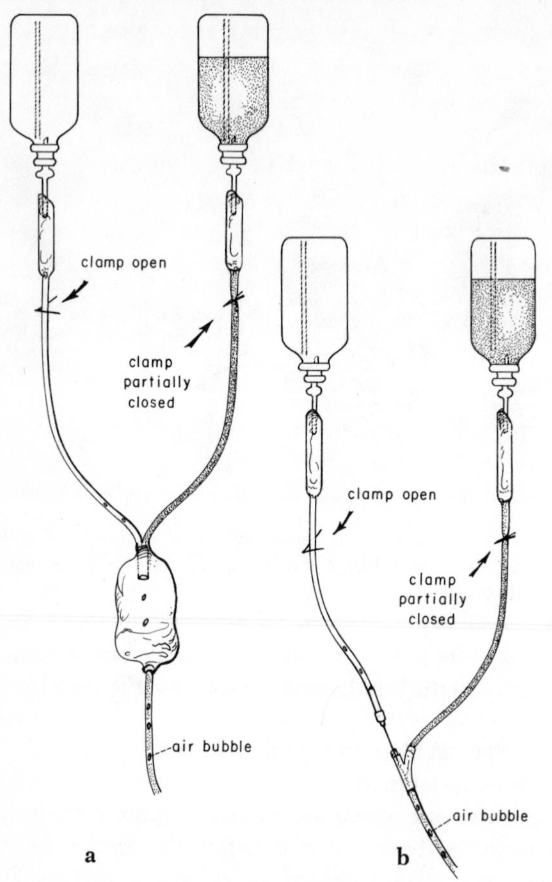

FIG. 22. (a) Bottle runs dry during simultaneous infusion of fluids through Y-type administration set. Pressure below the partially constricted clamp is less than atmospheric, allowing air from the empty bottle (atmospheric) to enter infusion.
(b) Secondary infusion piggybacked through injection site of a primary intravenous set. Lacking an automatic shut-off valve, air from the empty container will enter the circulation. The same principle is involved as in the Y-type set up.

on the infusion side. Recurrent small air bubbles are constantly aspirated into the flowing solution and on into the venous system. The introduction of air may be prevented by running one solution at a time. Vigilance is imperative if solutions are ordered to run simultaneously. The tubing must be clamped completely off before the solution bottle is allowed to empty [12].

This same principle is involved in the piggyback setup for secondary infusions. The potential danger of air embolism exists whenever solutions from two vented sets run simultaneously through a common needle.

All connections of an infusion set must be tight. Any faulty opening or defective hole in the set allows air to be emitted into the flowing solution. If a stopcock is used, the outlets not in use must be completely shut off.

The regulating clamp on the infusion set should be located no higher than the chest level of the patient. Since the pressure exerted by the blood on the venous wall will normally raise a column of water from 4 to 11 cm above the heart, a restricting clamp placed above this point will result in a negative pressure in the tubing [9]. If great enough, the pressure can suck air into the flowing solution should a loose connection or a faulty opening exist between the clamp and the needle [9]. The lower the clamp, the greater the chance of any existing defect to occur above the clamp, where positive pressure could force the solution to leak out [12].

An infusion set long enough to drop below the extremity gives added protection against air's being drawn into the vein should the infusion bottle empty. Inlying pressure pumps on administration sets should be kept filled at all times. Manual compression of an empty chamber will force air into the blood stream.

OCCURRENCE OF AN AIR EMBOLISM. The nurse should be familiar with the symptoms associated with air embolism which arise from sudden vascular collapse: cyanosis, drop in blood pressure, weak rapid pulse, rise in venous pressure, and loss of consciousness. If an air embolism occurs the patient should be turned on his left side with his head down [9]. This causes the air to rise in the right atrium preventing it from entering the pulmonary artery. Oxygen is administered and the physician notified.

Pulmonary edema

Overloading the circulation is a real hazard to the elderly patient and to those with impaired renal and cardiac function. Fluids too rapidly infused increase the venous pressure with the possibility of cardiac dilatation and subsequent pulmonary edema.

PREVENTIVE MEASURES. Measures should be taken to prevent pulmonary edema.

1. Infusions should be maintained at the flow rate prescribed.
2. Positive pressure should never be applied by the nurse to infuse solutions. If the patient requires fluids at such rapidity that positive pressure is required, it then becomes the physician's responsibility.
3. Solutions not infused within the 24-hour period ordered should be discarded and not infused with the following day's solutions. Fluids administered in excess of the quantity ordered can overtax the homeostatic controls, increasing the danger of pulmonary edema.
4. The attending nurse must be alert to any signs or symptoms significant of circulatory overloading. Venous dilatation, with engorged neck veins, increased blood pressure, and a rise in venous pressure, should alert the nurse to the danger of pulmonary edema. Rapid respiration and shortness of breath may occur. The infusion should be slowed to a minimum rate and the physician notified. Raising the patient to a sitting position may facilitate breathing.

Speed shock

Speed shock is the term used to denote the systemic reaction which occurs when a substance foreign to the body is rapidly introduced into the circulation. The rapid injection of a drug permits its concentration in the plasma to reach toxic proportions, flooding the organs rich in blood, the heart and the brain. As a result, syncope, shock, and cardiac arrest may occur [1].

PREVENTIVE MEASURES. Certain precautions can minimize the potential danger of speed shock.

1. Controlled volume infusion sets give added protection by preventing large quantities of fluid from being accidentally infused. These sets control the volume from 10 to 100 ml.
2. The pediatric-type infusion sets, by reducing the size of the drop, provide greater accuracy, thereby reducing the risk of rapid administration. They are valuable when solutions containing potent drugs must be maintained at a minimum rate of flow.
3. An extra clamp ensures greater safety should the initial clamp on the infusion set let go.
4. Upon initiating the infusion, ensure the solution is flowing freely before adjusting the rate; movement of a needle in which the aperture is partially obstructed by the wall of the vein could cause an increase in the flow contributing to the danger of speed shock.

REFERENCES

1. Adriani, J. Venipuncture. *American Journal of Nursing* 62:66–70, 1962.
2. Bard, C. R., Inc. *An Outline for the Use of IV Placement Units.* Murray Hill, N.J., 1970. Pp. 8, 9.
3. Druskin, M. S., and Siegel, P. D. Bacterial contamination of indwelling intravenous polyethylene catheters. *Journal of the American Medical Association* 185:966–968, 1963.
4. Editorial. Thrombophlebitis following intravenous infusions. *Lancet* 1:907–909, 1960.
5. Fonkalsrud, E. W., Pederson, B. M., et al. Reduction of infusion thrombophlebitis with buffered glucose solutions. *Surgery* 63:280–284, 1968.
6. Hickan, J. B., and Sieker, H. O. Pulmonary embolism and infarction. *DM: Disease-a-Month.* Chicago: Year Book Medical Publishers, Jan. 1959.

7. McNair, T. J., and Dudley, H. A. F. The local complications of intravenous therapy. *Lancet* 2:365–368, 1959.
8. Mavor, G. E., and Galloway, J. M. D. The ileofemoral venous segment as a source of pulmonary emboli. *Lancet* 1:873, 1967.
9. Metheny, N. M., and Snively, W. D., Jr. *Nurses' Handbook of Fluid Balance*. Philadelphia: Lippincott, 1967. Pp. 137–140.
10. Moran, J. M., Atwood, R. P., and Rowe, M. I. A clinical and bacteriologic study of infections associated with venous cutdown. *New England Journal of Medicine* 272:554–556, 1965.
11. Pfizer Laboratories. Intravenous technique. *Spectrum* 9:2–5, 1965.
12. Tarail, R. Practice of fluid therapy. *Journal of the American Medical Association* 171:45–49, 1950.
13. Vere, D. W., Sykes, C. H., and Armitage, P. Venous thrombosis during dextrose infusion. *Lancet* 2:627–630, 1960.
14. Williams, J. T., and Moravec, D. F. *Intravenous Therapy*. Hammond, Ind.: Clissold Publishing, 1967. P. 59.

8. Fundamental Aspects of Fluid and Electrolyte Metabolism

OVER THE PAST TEN YEARS our knowledge of fluid and electrolyte balance has increased to the extent that we now recognize an imbalance as a threat to life. With this increased knowledge has come an increase in the nurse's responsibility in parenteral therapy. Not only is accurate recording of the patient's intake and output important, but also the ability to recognize symptoms of imbalance; prompt recognition of an imbalance may indicate adjustment in therapy which may be crucial to the safety of the patient.

Today electrolyte therapy is used extensively. About 70 percent of all fluids administered contain some electrolytes. A survey done at the Massachusetts General Hospital in 1967 by S. Shamsi, Staff Pharmacist, revealed that 48 percent of 1911 solutions administered intravenously were electrolyte solutions. Of the remaining 52 percent of nonelectrolyte solutions, potassium chloride was added to about 20 percent.

Electrolyte therapy is often a lifesaving procedure; its safe and successful administration is essential. Knowledge of the fundamentals of fluid and electrolyte metabolism contributes to safe electrolyte therapy. This knowledge alerts the nurse to (1) the necessity for accurate fluid and electrolyte administration, (2) the potential dangers of electrolyte therapy, and (3) a change in the patient's condition which could alter the therapy prescribed.

Abnormalities of body fluid and electrolyte metabolism present certain therapeutic problems. When the mechanisms normally regulating fluid volume, electrolyte composition, and osmolality are impaired, therapy becomes complicated. An understanding of these metabolic abnormalities enables the nurse to understand the problems involved. Such problems exist in patients with renal insufficiency, adrenal insufficiency, adrenal hyperactivity, and other kinds of impaired organ function. For example, correction of a severe potassium deficit resulting from vomiting and diarrhea presents a problem in the dehydrated patient. Potassium replacement is imperative. However, potassium administered to patients with renal insufficiency results in potassium toxicity; the kidneys are unable to excrete electrolytes. The adverse effects of excess potassium on the heart muscle are arrhythmia and heart block. The nurse must recognize the importance of (1) hydrating the patient before potassium can be administered safely, and (2) watching for diminished diuresis which could necessitate a change in therapy. Once antidiuresis occurs the potassium infusion must be interrupted and the physician notified.

Therapeutic problems also exist in patients with impaired liver function. Gastric replacement is necessary when there has been an excessive loss of gastric fluid. Most deficits caused by gastric suction, unless severe, are treated with 0.85 percent sodium chloride (NaCl) in 5 percent dextrose in water (D/W). However, severe loss may call for gastric replacement solutions containing ammonium chloride, which can be potentially dangerous when administered to patients with impaired liver function. Ammonium chloride administered to a patient with severe liver damage may result in ammonia intoxication because of the liver's inability to convert ammonia to hydrogen ion and urea.

These examples illustrate the role that knowledge of fluid and electrolyte metabolism plays in contributing to safe and successful therapy in the critically ill patient.

FLUID CONTENT OF THE BODY

The total body water content of an individual varies with age, weight, and sex. The amount of water is dependent on the amount of body fat. Body fat is essentially water-free; the greater the fat content, the less the water content. In a normal male with an average amount of fat, the water weight is about 60 percent of the body weight. In a female, because of the normally larger degree of body fat, the proportion of water weight to body weight is less, about 54 percent of body weight.

COMPARTMENTS

The total body fluid is functionally divided into two main compartments: the intracellular and the extracellular compartments. The intracellular compartment consists of the fluid inside the cells and comprises about two thirds or 40 percent of the body fluid. The extracellular compartment consists of fluid outside the body cells—the plasma representing 5 percent of the body weight and the interstitial fluid (fluid in tissues) representing 15 percent of body fluid. See Table 3 for a schematic representation of compartments.

In newborn infants the proportion is approximately three fifths intracellular and two fifths extracellular. This ratio changes and reaches the adult level by the time the infant is about 30 months old.

There is one additional compartment, the transcellular compartment. The transcellular fluid is the product of cellular metabolism and consists of secretions such as gastrointestinal secretions and urine. Analysis of these secretions may assist the physician in tracing lost electrolytes and prescribing proper fluid and electrolyte replacement. Excessive fluid and electrolyte loss must be replaced to maintain fluid and electrolyte balance in the two main compartments. The amount of body water loss is easily computed by weighing the patient and noting loss of weight: 1 liter of body water is equivalent to 1 kg or 2.2 pounds body weight. Up to 5 percent weight loss in a child or

TABLE 3. Total Body Water Composition

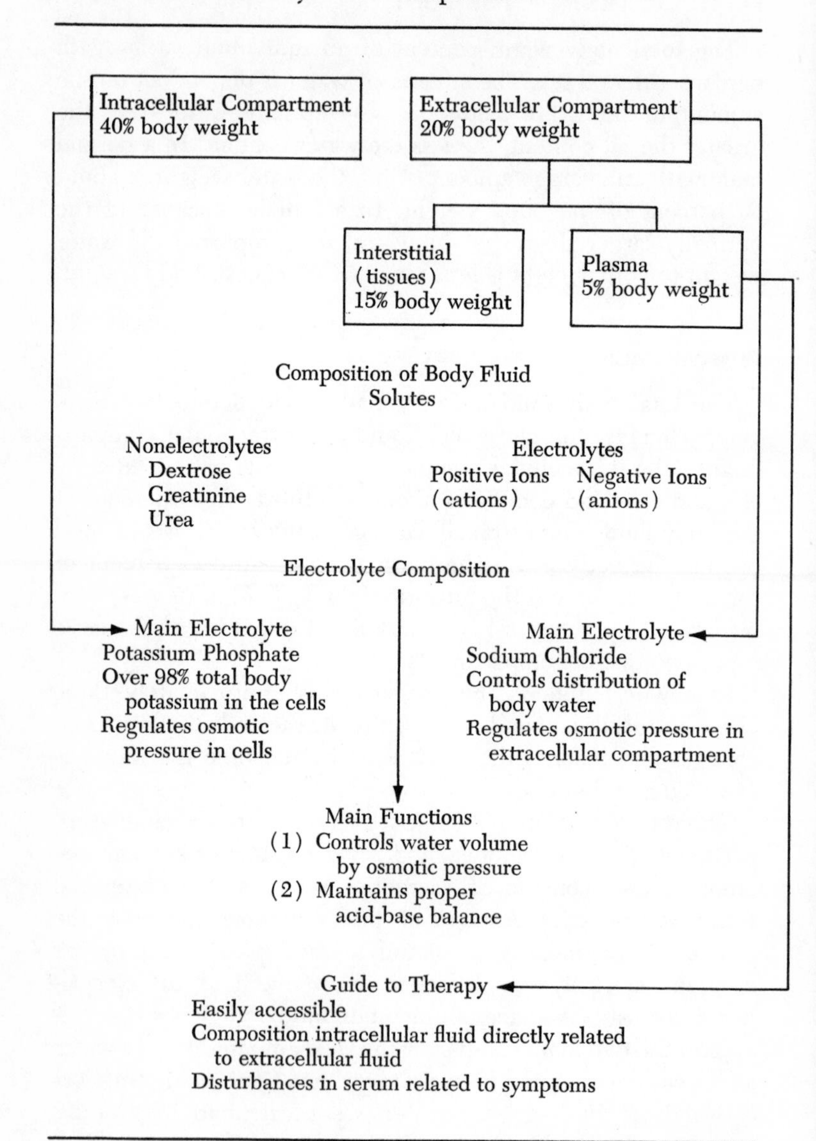
Intracellular Compartment
40% body weight
Extracellular Compartment
20% body weight
Interstitial
(tissues)
15% body weight
Plasma
5% body weight
Composition of Body Fluid
Solutes
Nonelectrolytes
Dextrose
Creatinine
Urea
Electrolytes
Positive Ions
(cations)
Negative Ions
(anions)
Electrolyte Composition
Main Electrolyte
Potassium Phosphate
Over 98% total body potassium in the cells
Regulates osmotic pressure in cells
Main Electrolyte
Sodium Chloride
Controls distribution of body water
Regulates osmotic pressure in extracellular compartment
Main Functions
(1) Controls water volume by osmotic pressure
(2) Maintains proper acid-base balance
Guide to Therapy
Easily accessible
Composition intracellular fluid directly related to extracellular fluid
Disturbances in serum related to symptoms

adult may signify moderate fluid volume deficit—over 5 percent may indicate severe fluid volume deficit [7]. Weight changes are also valuable as indicators of body water gains—acute weight gain may indicate water excess.

COMPOSITION OF BODY FLUID

The body fluid contains two types of solutes (dissolved substances): the electrolytes and the nonelectrolytes (see Table 3). The *nonelectrolytes* are molecules which do not break into particles in solution but remain intact. They consist of (1) dextrose, (2) urea, and (3) creatinine.

Electrolytes are molecules which break into electrically charged particles called ions. The ion carrying a positive charge is called a cation, the ion with a negative charge, an anion. Potassium chloride is an electrolyte which, dissolved in water, yields potassium cations (K^+) and chloride anions (Cl^-). Chemical balance is always maintained; the total number of positive charges equals the total number of negative charges. The quantity of charges and their concentration is expressed as milliequivalents (mEq) per liter of fluid. As the number of negative charges must equal the number of positive charges for chemical balance, the mEq of cations must equal the mEq of anions [2] (see Table 4).

TABLE 4. Plasma Electrolytes Illustrate That Total mEq of Cations Must Equal Total mEq of Anions

Cations	mEq/L	Anions	mEq/L
Na^+	142	HCO_3^-	24
K^+	5	Cl^-	105
Ca^{++}	5	HPO_4^{--}	2
Mg^{++}	2	SO_4^{--}	1
		Organic Acid−	6
		Proteinate−	16
Total	154	Total	154

SOURCE: Baxter Laboratories [2].

Electrolyte composition

Each fluid compartment has its own electrolyte composition (see Table 3). The extracellular compartment (plasma and interstitial fluid) contains a high concentration of sodium, chloride, and bicarbonate and a low concentration of potassium. The composition of the intracellular fluid is quite different; the concentrations of potassium, magnesium, and phosphate are high whereas the sodium and chloride concentrations are relatively low.

Electrolyte composition of the intracellular fluid is in part related to electrolyte composition in the plasma and interstitial fluids. Disturbances in the extracellular fluid are reflected in the patient's symptoms. These facts, combined with the accessibility of plasma, make the analysis of plasma a valuable guide to therapy. Occasionally, however, the electrolyte determination of plasma may be misleading. For example, concentration of potassium in plasma may be high while there is a body deficit. This surplus is due to the shift of potassium from intracellular to extracellular fluid in the process of large potassium losses through the kidneys. Determination of plasma sodium may also present a false picture. In the case of an edematous cardiac patient, the plasma concentration may be low in spite of excess body sodium. This is due to the fact that total body sodium is equal to the sum of the products of volume times concentration in the various compartments.

Electrolytes serve two main purposes: (1) to act in controlling body water volume by osmotic pressure, and (2) to maintain the proper acid-alkaline balance of the body.

Osmolality. Osmolality is the total solute concentration and reflects the relative water and total solute concentration since it is expressed per liter of serum. The osmotic pressure is determined by the number of solutes in solution. If the extracellular fluid contains a relatively large number of dissolved particles and the intracellular fluid contains a small amount of dissolved particles, the osmotic pressure would cause water to pass from the less concentrated to the more concentrated. Therefore fluid from the intracellular compartment would pass into the extracellular compartment until the concentration became equal.

The unit of osmotic pressure is the osmole and the values are expressed in milliosmoles (mOsm). Normal blood plasma has an osmolality of 290 mOsm. The determination of serum osmolality is sometimes used to detect dehydration or overhydration. Because sodium chloride is the principal solute in the extracellular fluid, the osmolality reading usually parallels the sodium reading or is very close to 2 times the serum sodium plus 10. Therefore measurement of sodium concentration also indicates the water needs of the body. At times the osmolality reading may falsely indicate dehydration. Because the osmolality is the total solute concentration, nonelectrolytes are included in the reading. An elevated blood urea can therefore increase the osmolality without exerting osmotic pressure. A determination of the blood urea nitrogen (BUN) may apply a correction to the osmolality reading in cases of increased serum urea.

Acid–alkaline balance

The alkalinity or acidity of a solution depends on the degree of hydrogen ion concentration. An increase in the hydrogen ions results in a more acid solution, a decrease in a more alkaline solution. Acidity is expressed by the symbol pH, which refers to the amount of hydrogen ion concentration. A solution having a pH of 7 is regarded as neutral.

The extracellular fluid has a pH ranging from 7.35 to 7.45 and is thus slightly alkaline. When the pH of the blood is higher than 7.45, an alkaline condition exists; when lower than 7.35, an acid condition exists.

The biological fluids, both extracellular and intracellular, contain a buffer system which maintains the proper acid–alkaline balance. This buffer system consists of fluid with salts of a weak acid or weak base. A base or hydroxide neutralizes the effect of an acid. These weak acids and bases maintain pH values by soaking up surplus ions or releasing them; acids yield hydrogen ions, bases accept hydrogen ions.

The carbonic acid–sodium bicarbonate system is the most important buffer system in the extracellular compartment. The normal ratio is 1 part of carbonic acid to 20 parts of base bicarbonate which represents 1.33 mEq of carbonic acid to 27 mEq of base bicarbonate [7].

Acid–base imbalance

Acid–base imbalances are normally the result of an excess or a deficit in either base bicarbonate or carbonic acid. Deviations of pH from 7.35 to 7.45 are combated by the buffer system and by the respiratory and renal regulatory mechanisms. There are two types of disturbance that can affect the acid–base balance: respiratory and metabolic. Refer to Table 5 for a diagrammatic presentation of the material that follows.

RESPIRATORY DISTURBANCES. Respiratory disturbances affect the carbonic side of the balance by increasing or decreasing the carbonic acid; when carbon dioxide unites with the extracellular fluid, carbonic acid is produced.

Respiratory alkalosis is caused when excess carbon dioxide is exhaled during rapid or deep breathing. Carbonic acid is depleted due to the carbon dioxide loss. Respiratory alkalosis may occur as the result of emotional disturbances, such as anxiety and hysteria, and also from lack of oxygen or fever [6].

Symptoms are convulsions, tetany, and unconsciousness. Laboratory determination of urinary pH is above 7, plasma bicarbonate below 25 mEq per liter [7]. The body attempts to restore the ratio to normal by depressing the bicarbonate so as to compensate for the deficit in the carbonic acid.

Respiratory acidosis occurs when exhalation of CO_2 is depressed; the excess retention of CO_2 increases the carbonic acid. It may occur in conditions that interfere with normal breathing: emphysema, asthma, and pneumonia [6].

Symptoms are weakness, disorientation, depressed breathing, and coma. The urine pH is below 6 and the plasma bicarbonate is above 29 mEq per liter. The increase of the bicarbonate is due to the body's attempt to restore the carbonic acid–bicarbonate ratio [7].

METABOLIC DISTURBANCES. Metabolic disturbances affect the bicarbonate side of the balance. Kidney function controls the bicarbonate concentration by regulating the amount of cations (hydrogen, ammonium, and potassium) in exchange for sodium ions to combine with the reabsorbed bicarbonate in the distal tubular lumen. As hydrogen ions are excreted, bicarbonate is generated, maintaining the proper acid–base balance of the blood. Ammonia excretion is increased in response to a high acidity; bicarbonate replaces the ammonia.

Metabolic alkalosis is a condition associated with excess bicarbonate. This condition occurs when there is loss of chloride. Chloride and bicarbonate are both anions, which must equal the total number of cations. When the chloride anions are lost, the deficit must be made up by an equal number of anions to maintain electrolyte equilibrium; bicarbonate increases in compensation and alkalosis occurs.

Metabolic alkalosis is also associated with decreased levels of intracellular potassium. Potassium escapes from the cell into the extracellular fluid and is lost through the transcellular fluid. When body potassium is lost, the shift of the sodium and hydrogen ions from the extracellular fluid causes alkalosis, while the increase of hydrogen ions in the intracellular fluid causes acidosis of the cells.

Muscular hyperactivity, tetany, and depressed respiration are symptoms of metabolic alkalosis. The muscular hyperactivity and the tetany are symptoms of the deficit in ionized calcium which exists in alkalosis. Laboratory determinations are urinary pH above 7, plasma pH above 7.45, and bicarbonate above 29 mEq per liter in adults and 25 mEq per liter in children [7].

Treatment consists of the administration of solutions containing chloride to replace bicarbonate ions. Excess of bicarbonate ions is accompanied by potassium deficiency, so potassium must also be replaced.

TABLE 5. Acid–Base Imbalances

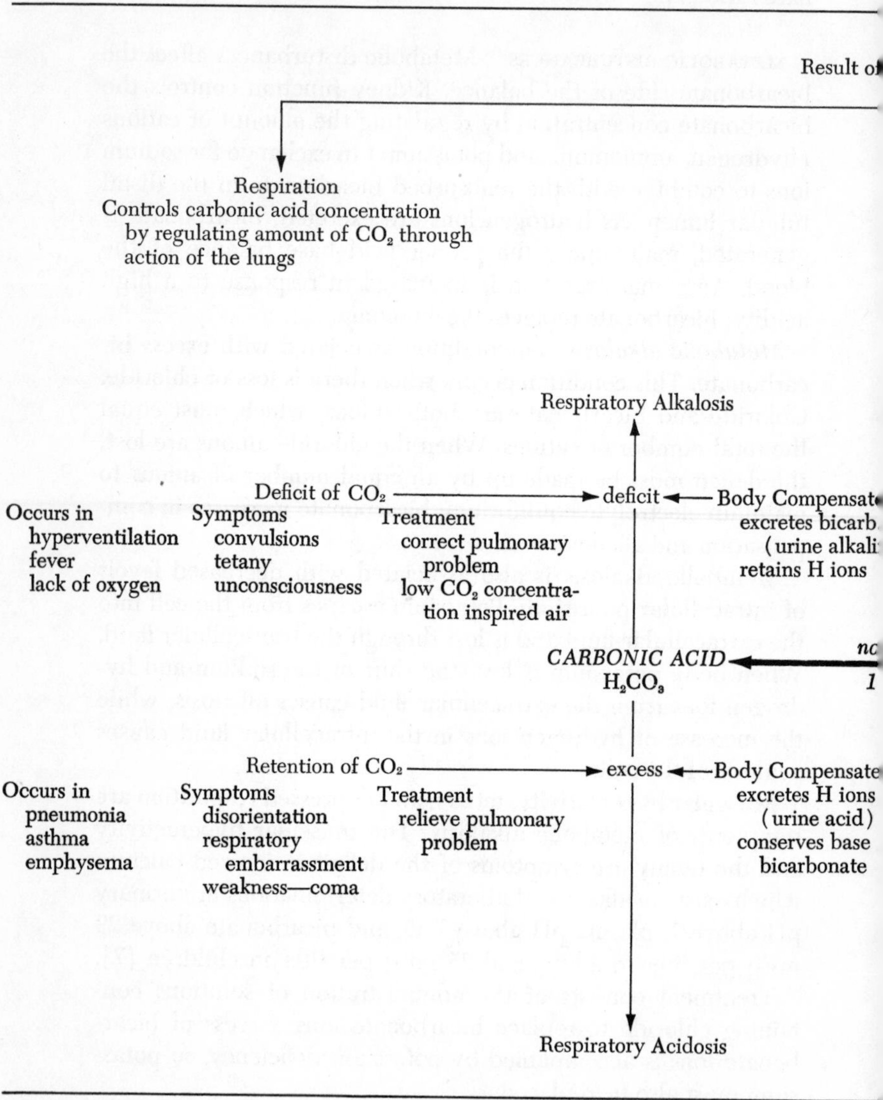

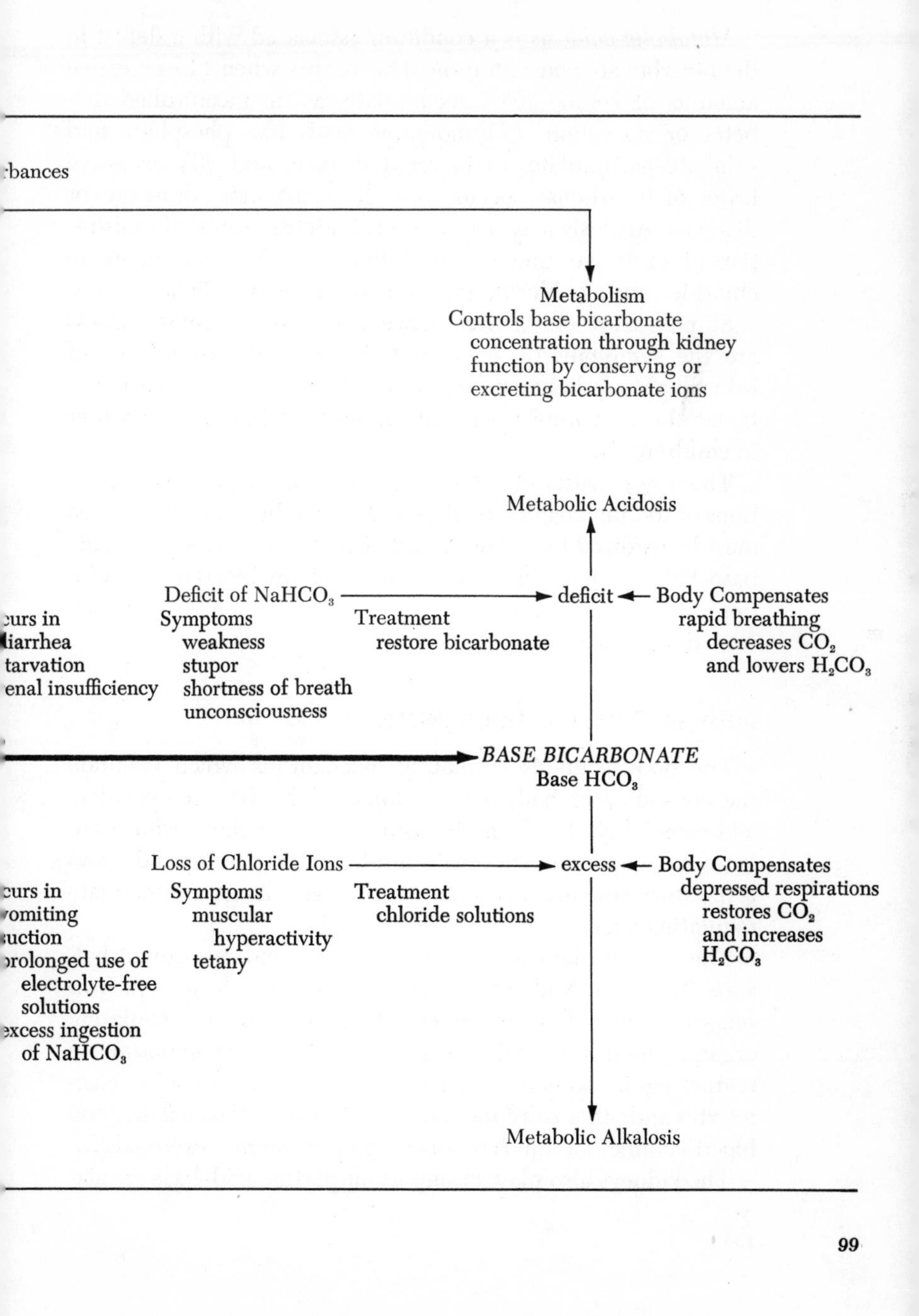
bances
Metabolism
Controls base bicarbonate concentration through kidney function by conserving or excreting bicarbonate ions
Metabolic Acidosis
Deficit of $NaHCO_3$
deficit
Body Compensates
rapid breathing
decreases CO_2
and lowers H_2CO_3
curs in
iarrhea
tarvation
enal insufficiency
Symptoms
weakness
stupor
shortness of breath
unconsciousness
Treatment
restore bicarbonate
BASE BICARBONATE
Base HCO_3
Loss of Chloride Ions
excess
Body Compensates
depressed respirations
restores CO_2
and increases
H_2CO_3
curs in
omiting
uction
rolonged use of
electrolyte-free
solutions
xcess ingestion
of $NaHCO_3$
Symptoms
muscular
hyperactivity
tetany
Treatment
chloride solutions
Metabolic Alkalosis

Metabolic acidosis is a condition associated with a deficit in the bicarbonate concentration. This occurs when (1) excessive amounts of ketone acids accumulate, as in uncontrolled diabetes or starvation, (2) inorganic acids like phosphate and sulphate accumulate, as in renal disease, and (3) excessive losses of bicarbonate occur from gastrointestinal drainage or diarrhea. Acidosis may occur also from intravenous administration of excessive amounts of sodium chloride or ammonium chloride causing chloride ions to flood the extracellular fluid.

Stupor, shortness of breath, weakness, and unconsciousness are the symptoms of acidosis. Laboratory determinations of urinary pH are below 6, plasma pH below 7.35, plasma bicarbonate below 25 mEq per liter in adults and 20 mEq per liter in children [7].

Therapy consists of increasing the bicarbonate level. Solutions of sodium lactate are often employed, but since lactate ion must be oxidized to carbon dioxide before it can affect the acid–base balance, it is advisable to use sodium bicarbonate solutions which are effective even when the patient is suffering from oxygen lack.

BODY REGULATING MECHANISMS

The body contains regulating mechanisms which maintain the constancy of body fluid volume, electrolyte composition, and osmolality. These mechanisms consist of the cardiovascular, renal, endocrine (adrenal, pituitary, and parathyroid), and respiratory systems. The kidneys, skin, and lungs are the main regulating agents [5].

The *kidney* plays a major role in fluid and electrolyte balance. To function adequately, the kidney depends upon its own soundness as well as on the coordination of all the regulating organs. The distal renal tubules in the kidney are important in regulating the body fluid. They selectively retain or reject electrolytes and other substances to maintain normal osmolality and blood volume; sodium is retained and potassium is excreted [2].

The kidneys also play an important part in acid–base regulation. The distal tubule has the ability to form ammonia and exchange hydrogen ion (in form of ammonia) for bicarbonate to maintain carbonic acid–bicarbonate ratio.

The *lungs* and the *skin* play an important role in fluid balance—the skin in loss of fluid through insensible perspiration and the lungs in fluid loss by expiration. It has been noted [3] that normal intake of 2500 ml from all sources will deliver a loss of about 1000 ml in breath and perspiration, 1400 ml in urine, and only 100 ml in feces.

The *cardiovascular system* maintains fluid balance by regulating the amount and composition of urine. Renal disease, cardiac failure, shock, postoperative stress, and alarm impair this regulating mechanism [5].

The adrenal glands influence the retention or excretion of sodium, potassium, and water. These glands secrete aldosterone, a hormone that increases the reabsorption of sodium from the renal tubules in exchange for potassium, thus maintaining normal sodium concentration [5]. Any stress, such as surgery, increases the secretion of aldosterone, thus increasing the reabsorption of sodium bicarbonate. Adrenal hyperactivity also increases the secretions of the hormone and causes excess sodium retention. Excessive loss of sodium occurs with adrenal insufficiency.

The *pituitary gland* is another important organ in the control of fluid and electrolyte balance. The posterior lobe of the pituitary releases antidiuretic hormone (ADH). This hormone inhibits diuresis by increasing water reabsorption in the distal tubule. "The release of ADH is influenced by the 'osmostat,' an auxiliary control located in the plexus of the internal carotid artery" [7]. Increased concentration of sodium in the extracellular fluid alerts the osmostat to signal the pituitary to release ADH. This hormone increases the reabsorption of water to dilute the sodium to the normal level of concentration. Increased body fluid osmolality, decreased body fluid volume, stress, and shock are conditions which increase hormone secretions. Increased body fluid volume, decreased osmolality, and alcohol inhibit the hormone secretions.

The *pulmonary system* regulates acid–base balance by controlling the concentration of carbonic acid through exhalation or retention of carbon dioxide.

ELECTROLYTES OF BIOLOGICAL FLUIDS

POTASSIUM

Potassium is one of the most important electrolytes in the body. An excess or deficiency of potassium can cause serious impairment of body function and even result in death.

It is the main electrolyte in the intracellular compartment, which houses over 98 percent of the body's total potassium. The healthy cell requires a high potassium concentration for cellular activity. When the cell dies, there is an exchange of potassium into the extracellular fluid with a transfer of sodium into the cell. This process also occurs to some degree when cellular metabolism is impaired, as in catabolism (breaking down) of cells from a crushing injury.

Plasma concentration of potassium is 4.0 to 5.5 mEq per liter. In the cell, the normal concentration is 115 to 150 mEq per liter of fluid. Variations from either of these levels can produce critical effects. High serum concentrations have an adverse effect on the heart muscle. At 7 mEq per liter an elevation of T waves in the electrocardiogram may be detected. With an extracellular level of 8 to 10 mEq per liter, arrhythmia and heart block may occur [1]. Hyperkalemia is the term which expresses serum potassium concentration above normal; hypokalemia, the serum potassium below normal.

HYPOKALEMIA. Hypokalemia (serum potassium below 4 mEq per liter) may result when any one of the following conditions occurs: (1) total body potassium is below normal, (2) concentration of potassium in cells is below normal, or (3) concentration of potassium in serum is below normal [4].

These conditions are often caused by variations in the intake or output of potassium. A decreased intake of potassium from prolonged fluid therapy (lacking potassium replacement) may result in hypokalemia. It may also occur during a "starvation diet," as the kidneys do not normally conserve potassium. An increased loss of potassium usually results from polyuria, vomiting, gastric suction (prolonged), diarrhea, and steroid therapy [4].

On the other hand, these conditions of potassium deficiency may be unrelated to intake and output. They can be caused by a sudden shift of potassium from extracellular fluid to intracellular fluid, such as that occurring from (1) anabolism (building up of cells), (2) healing process, or (3) the use of insulin and glucose in the treatment of diabetic acidosis [4]. The shifts resulting from anabolism and healing processes are not usually of severe consequence unless accompanied by intervening factors. In the treatment of diabetic acidosis, the potassium shift may occur suddenly with grave consequences. When cells are anabolized, potassium shifts into the cells. During the use of glucose in the treatment of diabetic acidosis, the glucose in the cells is quickly metabolized into glycogen for storage, causing a sudden shift of potassium from the extracellular fluid to the intracellular fluid [4]. This process results in hypokalemia.

The signs and symptoms of hypokalemia are malaise, skeletal and smooth muscle atonia, apathy, muscular cramps, and postural hypotension. Treatment consists of administration of potassium orally or parenterally.

HYPERKALEMIA. Hyperkalemia may result from renal failure with potassium retention or from excessive or rapid administration of potassium in fluid therapy. It may also occur in conditions unrelated to retention or excessive intake. A sudden shift of potassium from intracellular to extracellular fluid results when catabolism of cells takes place, as in a crushing injury; potassium shifts from cells to plasma.

The signs and symptoms of hyperkalemia are similar to those of hypokalemia. In addition to those signs already listed, the patient may experience tingling or numbness in extremities, and the heart rate may be slow. Potassium level above 5.5 mEq per liter confirms the diagnosis.

Treatment consists of stopping the potassium intake. Dialysis may be necessary for a long-term renal problem. If the cause is a shift of potassium from cells to plasma, glucose and insulin therapy may be used.

Sodium

Sodium is the main electrolyte in the extracellular fluid; its normal concentration is 135 to 142 mEq per liter of plasma. The main role of sodium is to control the distribution of water throughout the body and to maintain a normal fluid balance. Alterations in sodium concentration markedly influence the fluid volume: the loss or gain of sodium is accompanied by loss of water and dehydration or retention of fluid.

The body, by regulating the urinary output, normally maintains a constant fluid volume and isotonicity of the plasma. The urinary output is controlled by ADH, secreted by the pituitary gland. If a hypotonic concentration results from a low sodium concentration, the fluid is drawn from the plasma into the cells. Nature attempts to correct this process; the pituitary inhibits ADH and diuresis results with a loss of extracellular fluid. This loss of fluid increases sodium concentration to a normal level.

If a hypertonic concentration results from increased concentration of extracellular sodium, fluid is drawn from the cells. Again nature reacts, and the pituitary is stimulated to secrete ADH. This causes a retention of fluid diluting sodium to normal concentration.

Therefore increased sodium concentration stimulates the production of ADH, with retention of water thus diluting sodium to the normal level; a decrease in sodium concentration inhibits the production of ADH, resulting in a loss of water which raises the concentration of sodium to the normal level.

In the kidneys sodium is reabsorbed in exchange for potassium. Therefore with an increase in sodium there is loss of potassium; with a loss of sodium there is an increase in potassium.

A *sodium deficit* may be present when plasma sodium falls below 135 mEq per liter. It is caused by (1) excessive sweating with large intake of water by mouth (salt is lost and fluid increased, thus reducing sodium concentration), (2) excessive infusion of nonelectrolyte fluids, (3) gastrointestinal suction plus water by mouth, and (4) adrenal insufficiency, which causes large loss of electrolytes.

The symptoms of a sodium deficit are apprehension, abdominal cramps, diarrhea, and convulsions.

Dehydration results from loss of sodium and leads to peripheral circulatory failure. When sodium and water are lost from the plasma, the body attempts to replace them by a transfer of sodium and water from the interstitial fluid. Eventually the water will be drawn from the cells and circulation will fail; plasma volume will not be sustained [1].

Sodium excess may be present when the plasma sodium rises above 145 mEq per liter. Its causes are (1) excessive infusions of saline, (2) diarrhea, (3) insufficient water intake, (4) diabetes mellitus, and (5) tracheobronchitis (excess loss of water from lungs because of rapid breathing).

The symptoms of sodium excess are dry sticky mucous membranes, oliguria, excitement, and convulsions.

Calcium

Calcium is an electrolyte constituent of the plasma which is present in concentration of about 5 mEq per liter. Calcium serves several purposes. It plays an important role in formation and function of bones and teeth. As ionized calcium, it is involved in (1) normal clotting of the blood and (2) regulation of neuromuscular irritability.

The parathyroid gland, located within the thyroid gland, controls calcium metabolism. The parathyroid hormone, acting on the kidneys and bones, regulates the concentration of ionized calcium in the extracellular fluid. Impairment of this regulatory mechanism alters the calcium concentration. Hyperparathyroidism causes an elevation in the serum calcium and a decrease in the phosphate.

Calcium deficit may occur in patients with diarrhea or with problems in gastrointestinal absorption, in extensive infections of the subcutaneous tissue, and in burns [7]. This deficiency can result in muscle tremors and cramps, in excessive irritability, and even in convulsions.

Calcium ionization is influenced by pH; it is decreased in alkalosis and increased in acidosis. With no loss of calcium a patient in alkalosis may develop symptoms of calcium deficit: muscle cramps, tetany, and convulsions. This is due to the decreased ionization of calcium caused by the elevated pH.

A patient in acidosis may have a calcium deficit with no symptoms because the acid pH has caused an increased ionization of available calcium. Symptoms of calcium deficit may appear if acidosis is converted to alkalosis.

Other electrolytes

Magnesium's primary role is in enzyme activity, contributing to the metabolism of both carbohydrates and proteins. Its serum concentration is 1.7 to 2.3 mEq per liter. A deficit in magnesium is not common but may occur from impaired gastrointestinal absorption.

Chloride, the chief anion of the extracellular fluid, has a plasma concentration of 100 to 106 mEq per liter. A deficiency of chloride leads to a deficiency of potassium and vice versa. There is also a loss of chloride with a loss of sodium, but because this loss can be compensated for by an increase in bicarbonate, the proportion will differ [2].

Phosphate is the chief anion of the intracellular fluid; its normal level in plasma is 1.7 to 2.3 mEq per liter.

REFERENCES

1. Abbott Laboratories. *Fluid and Electrolytes.* North Chicago, Ill., 1960. Pp. 6–26.
2. Baxter Laboratories, Division of Travenol Laboratories, Inc. *Fundamentals of Body Water and Electrolytes.* Morton Grove, Ill., 1967. Pp. 5, 35.

3. Burgess, R. E. Fluids and electrolytes. *American Journal of Nursing* 65:90–95, 1965.
4. Crowell, C. E., and Staff of Educational Design, Inc., N.Y. Potassium imbalance. *American Journal of Nursing* 67:343, 1967.
5. McGaw Laboratories, Inc. *Guide to Parenteral Fluid Therapy*. Glendale, Cal., 1963. Pp. 7–13.
6. Mead Johnson & Company. *Fluid Therapy*. Parenteral Division, Evansville, Ind., 1957–1959. Pp. 107–113.
7. Metheny, N. M., and Snively, W. D., Jr. *Nurses' Handbook of Fluid Balance*. Philadelphia: Lippincott, 1967. Pp. 27, 30, 107, 212–213.

9.
Rationale of Fluid and Electrolyte Therapy

OBJECTIVES OF PARENTERAL THERAPY

Parenteral therapy has three main objectives: (1) to maintain daily requirements, (2) to restore previous losses, and (3) to replace present losses.

MAINTENANCE THERAPY

Maintenance therapy consists of provision of all the nutrient needs of the patient: water, electrolytes, dextrose, vitamins, and protein. Of these needs, water has the priority. The body may survive for a prolonged period without vitamins, dextrose, and protein, but without water, dehydration and death occur.

Water is needed by the body to replace the insensible loss which occurs with evaporation from the skin and evaporated moisture from the expired air. An average adult loses from 500 to 1000 ml of water per 24 hours through insensible loss [6]. The skin loss varies with the temperature and humidity.

Water must also be provided for kidney function; the amount needed depends upon the amount of waste products to be excreted as well as the concentrating ability of the kidneys [6]. Protein and salt increase the need for water.

Until 1925 parenteral fluids consisted solely of isotonic saline solutions [6]. Because water is hypotonic and cannot be given intravenously, salt was added to attain isotonicity. If given intravenously, distilled water causes hemolysis; the distilled water is drawn into the blood cells due to the greater solute concentration, causing them to swell and burst.

Because the normal plasma has an osmolality of 290 mOsm, parenteral fluids are considered isotonic, hypertonic, or hypotonic in their relation to plasma. Solutions with an osmolality significantly higher than 290 mOsm (+ 50 mOsm) are considered hypertonic, while those with an osmolality significantly lower than 290 mOsm (– 50 mOsm) are hypotonic [3]. For example, a solution of 5 percent dextrose in water (McGaw's solution) has an osmolality of 250 mOsm (isotonic), but by adding sodium chloride to 0.9 percent (310 mOsm), the osmolality of the solution is increased to 560 mOsm (hypertonic).

Parenteral solutions range largely from approximately half isotonic (0.45 percent sodium chloride) to 5 or 10 times isotonic (25 to 50 percent dextrose).

After 1925 glucose began to be used extensively to make water isotonic and to provide calories [6].

An individual's fluid requirements are based on age, height, weight, and amount of body fat. Because fat is water-free, a large amount of body fat contains a relatively low amount of water; as body fat increases, water decreases in inverse proportion to body weight [7]. The normal fluid and electrolyte requirements based on surface area have been found to be more constant than when expressed in terms of body weight. Many of the essential physiological processes such as heat loss, blood volume, organ size, and respiration have a direct relationship to the body surface area [8]. The fluid and electrolyte requirements are also in proportion to surface area, regardless of the age of the patient [8]. These requirements are based on square meter (m^2) of body surface and calculated for a 24-hour period. Nomograms are available for determining surface area (see Figure 23, page 112).

Balanced solutions are available for maintenance. An estimate is made of the average requirements of fluid and electrolytes in a healthy person and applied to the patient. The balanced solutions contain electrolytes in proportion to the daily needs of the patient, but not in excess of the body's tolerance, as long as adequate kidney function exists. When a patient's water needs are provided by these maintenance solutions, the daily need of sodium and potassium are also met. For maintenance, 1500 ml per square meter of body surface is administered over a 24-hour period [8].

Glucose, a necessary nutrient in maintenance therapy, has important functions. As it is converted into glycogen by the liver, it improves hepatic function. By supplying necessary calories for energy, it spares body protein and minimizes the development of ketosis occasioned by the oxidation of fat stores for essential energy in the absence of added glucose.

The basic daily caloric requirement of a 70 kg adult at rest is about 1600 calories. However, the administration of 100 gm of glucose a day is considered sufficient to help prevent ketosis [8]; 100 gm is contained in 2 liters of 5 percent dextrose in water or 1 liter of 10 percent dextrose in water.

Protein is another nutrient important to maintenance therapy. Though a patient may be adequately maintained on glucose, water, vitamins, and electrolytes over a limited time, protein may be required to replace normal protein losses over an extended period of time. It is necessary for cellular repair, healing of wounds, and synthesis of vitamins and some enzymes. The usual daily requirement for a healthy adult is 1 gm protein per kilogram of body weight [8]. Protein is available as amino acids; taken orally, it is broken down into amino acids before being absorbed into the blood.

Vitamins, though not nutrients in the true sense of the word, are necessary for the utilization of other nutrients. Vitamin C and the various B complex vitamins are the most frequently used in parenteral therapy. As these vitamins are water soluble, they are not retained by the body but lost through urinary excretion. Because of this loss, larger amounts are required parenterally to ensure adequate maintenance than may be required when administered orally. Vitamin B complex vitamins play an important role in the metabolism of carbohydrates

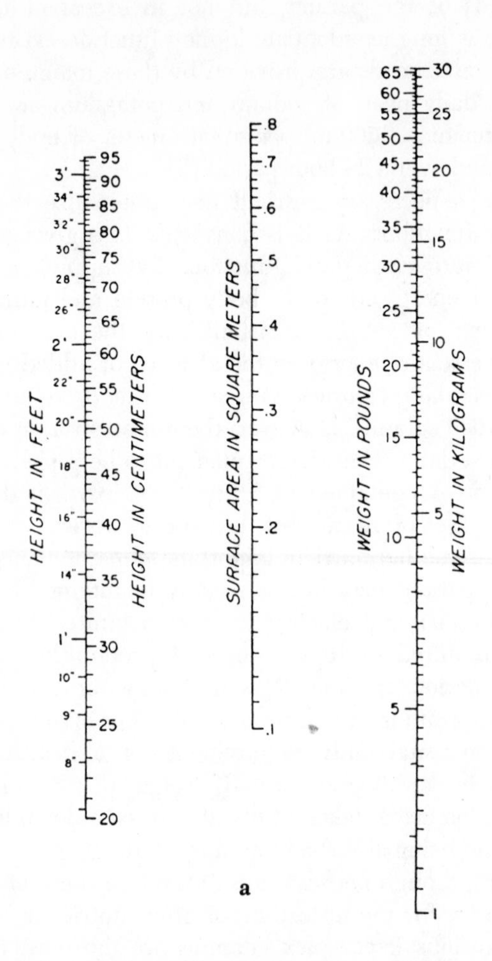

FIG. 23. Body surface area nomograms for (a) infants and young children, and (b) older children and adults [9]. To determine the surface area of the patient draw a straight line between the point representing his height on the left vertical scale to the point representing his weight on the right vertical scale. The point at which this line intersects the middle vertical scale represents the patient's surface area in square meters. (From Talbot et al. [9].)

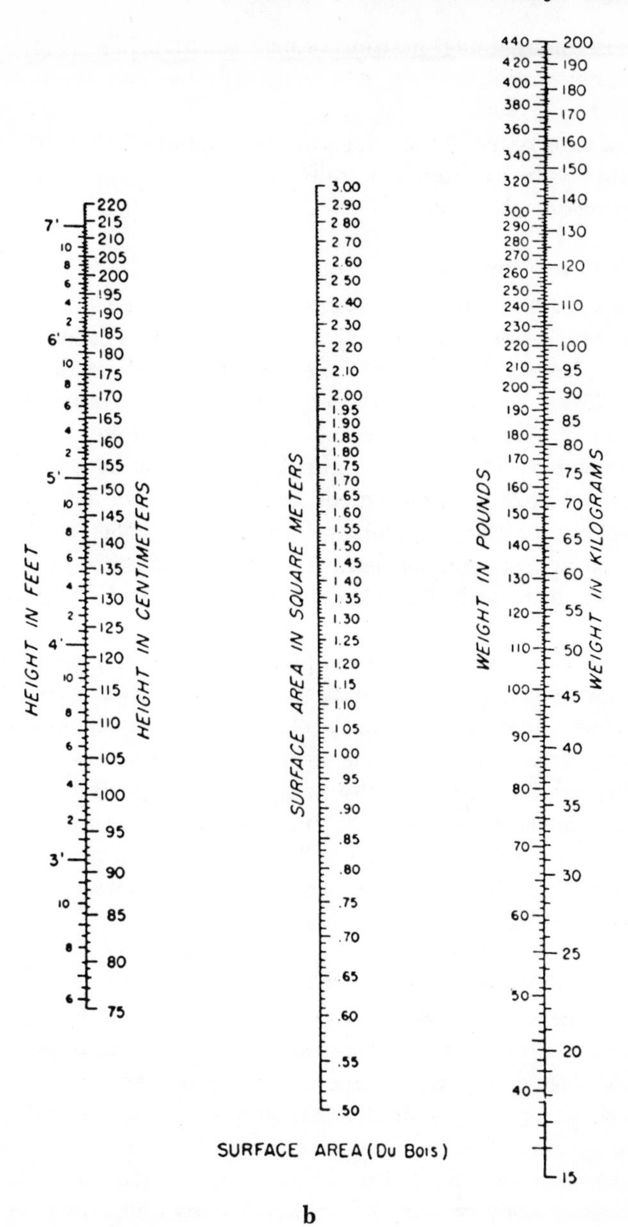
HEIGHT IN FEET
HEIGHT IN CENTIMETERS
SURFACE AREA IN SQUARE METERS
WEIGHT IN POUNDS
WEIGHT IN KILOGRAMS
SURFACE AREA (Du Bois)

b

and in maintaining gastrointestinal function. As vitamin C promotes wound healing, it is frequently used for the surgical patient.

Vitamins A and D are fat soluble vitamins, better retained by the body and not generally required by the patient on maintenance therapy.

Restoration of previous losses

Restoration of previous losses is essential when past maintenance has not been met—when the output has exceeded the intake. Severe dehydration may occur from failure to replace these losses. Therapy consists of replacing losses from previous deficits in addition to providing fluid and electrolytes for daily maintenance. The status of the kidneys must be considered before electrolyte replacement and maintenance can be initiated; urinary suppression may result from decreased fluid volume or renal impairment. A hydrating solution such as 5 percent dextrose in 0.2 percent (34.2 mEq) sodium chloride is administered. Urinary flow will be restored if the retention is functional. The patient must be rehydrated rapidly to establish an adequate urinary output. Only after kidney function is proved adequate can large electrolyte losses be replaced. Potassium chloride must be used with considerable caution and is considered potentially dangerous if administered when renal function is impaired. A buildup of potassium, due to the kidney's inability to excrete salts, can prove hazardous; arrhythmia and heart block can result from the effect of excess potassium on the heart muscle.

Replacement of present losses

Replacement of present losses of fluid and electrolytes is as necessary as daily maintenance and replacement of previous losses. The importance of accurate measurement of all intake and output cannot be underestimated as a means of calculating fluid loss. Fluid loss may also be estimated by determining loss of body weight; 1 liter of body water equals 1 kg or 2.2 pounds of body weight. An osmolality determination may indicate the water needs of the body. If necessary a corrective BUN may be done in conjunction with the osmolality.

The type of replacement is dependent on the type of fluid being lost. A choice of appropriate replacement solutions is available. Excessive loss of gastric fluid must be replaced by solutions resembling the fluid lost, such as gastric replacement solutions. Excessive loss of intestinal fluid must be replaced by an intestinal replacement fluid.

Examples of conditions that may result from current losses are alkalosis and acidosis (see Table 5, Chapter 8). *Alkalosis* may occur from an excessive loss of gastric fluid, either by vomiting or suction. Gastric juices, with a pH of 1 to 3, are the most acid of the body secretions [8]. Loss of excess chloride causes an increase in the bicarbonate ions; total anions must always equal total cations. The patient's respiration becomes slow and shallow; the body attempts to correct alkalosis by retaining CO_2. Because of the body's inability to ionize calcium in the presence of a high pH, muscular hyperactivity and tetany occur. The patient may become irritable, uncooperative, and disoriented.

Prompt recognition of symptoms is important for early treatment or for altering current treatment. Most alkalotic states secondary to gastric suction are corrected by sodium chloride and potassium chloride solutions. Special gastric replacement solutions are available. They contain ammonium chloride, which replaces the chloride without increasing the sodium. The hydrogen ions, liberated by urea in the conversion of ammonium chloride, correct alkalosis. These solutions, invaluable in certain conditions, can be potentially dangerous if given to patients with impaired liver or kidney function. Ammonia, metabolized by the liver, is converted into urea and hydrogen ion. If the liver fails to convert the ammonia to urea, ammonia retention and toxicity will result. Symptoms of ammonia toxicity include pallor, sweating, tetany, and coma, and may result in death.

Acidosis may occur when the excessive fluid loss is alkaline, as are intestinal secretions, bile, and pancreatic juices. Intestinal secretions contain large amounts of bicarbonate ions; with the loss of these ions, there is an increase in the chloride ions—and acidosis occurs. Symptoms include shortness of breath with rapid breathing (respiratory compensation to reduce CO_2 and correct acidosis). Weakness and coma occur. In order to replace lost alkaline secretions and correct acidosis, specific parenteral solutions containing base salts, such as sodium lactate or sodium bicarbonate, are employed.

ELECTROLYTE AND FLUID DISTURBANCES

Fluid and electrolyte imbalances occurring in the ill patient are serious complications which can threaten life. The correction of these imbalances is of vital concern to the welfare of the patient. A discussion follows of a few of the most common clinical cases in which fluid disturbances contribute to serious complications, with emphasis on physiological changes accompanying these imbalances and the parenteral therapy necessary to correct them.

PARENTERAL THERAPY FOR THE SURGICAL PATIENT

A knowledge of the endocrine response to stress assists the nurse in a better understanding of imbalances and problems associated with them. It also contributes to safe and successful parenteral therapy: The nurse knows what to expect, is alert to the possible dangers of imbalances, and recognizes early symptoms.

Endocrine response to stress

The endocrine homeostatic controls are affected by stress. At times stress from preoperative apprehension triggers an undesirable endocrine response, making it necessary to postpone an operation. Apprehension, pain, and duration and severity of trauma give rise to surgical stress and cause an increased endocrine response during the first 2 to 5 days following surgery. On the whole the stress reaction is normal and is nature's way of protecting the body from hypotension resulting from trauma and shock. Correction is often unnecessary and may, in fact, be harmful.

The two major endocrine homeostatic controls affected by stress are the pituitary gland and the adrenal gland (see Table 6). The posterior pituitary controls quantitative secretions of ADH (antidiuretic hormone); the anterior pituitary controls secretions of ACTH (adrenocorticotropic hormone). ACTH stimulates the adrenal gland to increase (1) mineralcorticoid secretions (aldosterone) and (2) glucocorticoid secretions (hydrocortisone) [8]. The adrenal medulla secretes vasopressors (epinephrine and norepinephrine) to help maintain the blood pressure.

A direct physiological effect is produced when stress increases the secretions of these various hormones. When the posterior pituitary increases ADH secretions, antidiuresis is effected, thus helping maintain blood volume. When the anterior pituitary increases ACTH secretions, the adrenal gland is stimulated to increase the secretions of aldosterone and hydrocortisone. These two adrenal hormones help maintain blood volume by (1) causing the retention of Na^+ and Cl^-, thereby causing water retention, and (2) promoting the excretion of K (loss of cellular K^+ causes loss of cellular water into extracellular space, where it is retained by ADH to maintain blood volume) [8].

Hydrocortisone also promotes the catabolism of protein to provide necessary amino acids for healing and stimulates the conversion of protein and fat to glucose for metabolism during the stress period. This metabolic activity may elevate the blood sugar, a finding which may mistakenly suggest diabetes mellitus. A drop in the eosinophil count indicates increased adrenal activity [8].

Fluid therapy

Accurate records of intake and output measurements are important for assessing the proper fluid requirements and pre-

TABLE 6. Endocrine Response to Stress

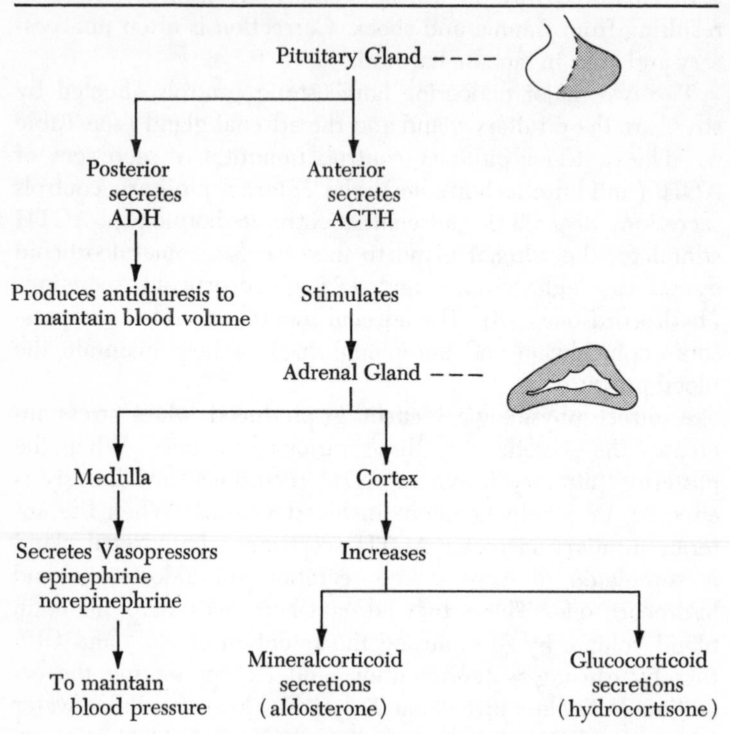

Retains Na and Cl causing water retention
Promotes excretion of potassium (loss of cellular K causes loss of cellular water into extravascular space where it is retained by ADH to increase the blood volume)

Hydrocortisone also
1. Promotes catabolism of protein providing amino acids for healing
2. Stimulates conversion of protein and fat to glucose for metabolizing during stress periods

Drop in eosinophil indicates increased adrenal activity.

venting serious fluid imbalances during the early postoperative period. The daily requirement of 1500 to 2000 ml varies with the patient's needs. Caution must be taken not to overhydrate the patient—the intake should be adequate but should not exceed the fluid losses.

We have seen how the adrenocortical secretions, increased by trauma and stress of surgery, cause some water and sodium retention. This retention may be severe enough to give a false picture of oliguria. Excessive quantities of nonelectrolyte solutions, such as 5 percent dextrose in water, administered at a time when antidiuresis is occurring may cause a serious fluid imbalance, hyponatremia.

Hyponatremia is a condition in which the serum sodium is less than the normal concentration in the serum. Water-yielding solutions, infused in excess of the body's tolerance, expand the extracellular compartment, lowering the electrolyte concentration. Water by the process of osmosis invades the cells with a resulting excess accumulation of intracellular fluid. Usually there is no edema, as edema is the result of an excess accumulation of fluid in the extracellular compartment [3].

Symptoms of water excess include confusion, hallucinations, delirium, weight gain, hyperventilation, muscular weakness, twitching, and convulsions. If these occur during the early postoperative stages, the nurse should suspect water excess. This is of particular concern in the young and the aged. Serious consequences, even death, can result.

Restricting the fluid intake may correct mild water excess, but for the more severe cases the administration of high concentrations of sodium chloride may be indicated. The electrolyte concentration of the plasma, increased by the concentrated saline, causes an increase in the osmotic pressure, drawing fluid from the cells for excretion by the kidneys.

Often parenteral therapy during the stress period consists of administering conservative amounts of 5 percent dextrose in water. As some sodium retention results from the endocrine response to stress, caution is taken to avoid administration of excessive quantities of saline at a time when there is an interference in the elimination of salt. During this early period, the physician frequently gives 5 percent dextrose in quarter or half strength saline to avoid sodium excess.

Sodium excess is a condition or state in which the serum sodium is higher than the normal concentration in the serum. This excess can cause (1) expanded extracellular fluid volume or edema and (2) possible disruption of cellular function (in potassium-depleted patients the sodium may replace the intracellular potassium).

Symptoms of sodium excess include flushed skin, elevation in temperature, dry sticky mucous membranes, thirst, and a decrease or absence of urinary output. Treatment consists of reducing the intake of salt and water and in promoting diuresis to eliminate the excess of salt and water from the plasma.

NUTRIENTS

CARBOHYDRATES. Carbohydrates provide an indispensable source of calories for the postoperative patient unable to receive oral sustenance. When carbohydrates are inadequate, the body will utilize its own fat to supply calories; the by-products are ketone bodies. These acid bodies neutralize bicarbonate and produce metabolic acidosis. The only by-products to be excreted in the utilization of carbohydrates are water and carbon dioxide.

Carbohydrates, by providing calories for essential energy, also reduce catabolism of protein. During the stress response the renal excretion of nitrogen (from the catabolism of protein) exceeds the intake. By reducing the protein breakdown, glucose helps prevent a negative nitrogen balance. The administration of as little as 100 gm of carbohydrate (2 liters of 5 percent glucose or 1 liter of 10 percent glucose) daily can reduce catabolism by as much as one half [8].

Carbohydrates do not provide adequate calories for the patient on prolonged therapy. One liter of 5 percent dextrose in water (McGaw's solution) provides 170 calories. Many liters, a volume too great for most patients to tolerate, would be required to provide a patient with 1600 calories. Greater concentrations of glucose, 20 percent and 50 percent, may be administered to provide calories for patients unable to tolerate large volumes of fluid (e.g., patients with renal insufficiency). The concentrated solutions must be administered slowly for utilization of the glucose to take place. Rapid administration results in diuresis; the concentrated glucose acts as a diuretic, drawing interstitial fluid into the plasma for excretion by the kidneys. Glucose may be administered to normal individuals at a maximum speed of about 0.5 gm per kilogram per hour without producing glycosuria [8].

Another condition, hyperinsulinism, may result from too rapid an infusion of hypertonic carbohydrate solutions. In response to the rise in blood sugar, the beta islet cells of the pancreas pour out extra insulin to metabolize the infused carbohydrates; termination of the infusion may leave excess insulin in the body causing such symptoms as nervousness, sweating, and weakness. Frequently after infusion of hypertonic dextrose, small amounts of isotonic dextrose solutions are administered to cover the excess insulin.

ALCOHOL. Alcohol solutions may be administered to the postoperative patient for nutritional and physiological benefits. Nutritionally the alcohol supplements calories provided by the glucose, 1 gm of ethyl alcohol yielding 6 to 8 calories [8]. Because alcohol is quickly and completely metabolized, it provides calories for essential energy, sparing fat and protein. Metabolized in preference to glucose, alcohol allows the infused glucose to be stored as glycogen.

Physiologically, alcohol produces a sedative effect, reducing pain; 200 to 300 ml of a 5 percent solution per hour produces sedation without intoxication in the average adult [8]. Alcohol also inhibits the secretion of ADH, promoting water excretion.

It is well to bear in mind that the solutions containing alcohol, particularly hypertonic solutions, can cause phlebitis. These solutions, if allowed to infiltrate, may cause tissue necrosis. The needle should be carefully inserted within the vein and inspected frequently to detect any infiltration.

AMINO ACIDS. Amino acids are beneficial to the surgical patient after the catabolic state has passed. They are usually used in conjunction with alcohol and glucose; alcohol and glucose provide calories for metabolism while the protein is made available for tissue repairs.

Before amino acids are administered, the patient should be questioned regarding allergies and the infusion should be started slowly and cautiously. Sometimes rapid infusion causes nausea, flushed face, and a feeling of warmth. Reducing the speed should alleviate these symptoms.

Commercial solutions containing alcohol, dextrose, and amino acids are available in varying strengths and caloric values. No solutions should be used which are cloudy or contain precipitate [2]. These solutions, once opened, must be used immediately. Storing a partially used bottle in the refrigerator for later use may provide a culture medium for the growth of bacteria. Use of such contaminated solutions has been known to lead to death.

POTASSIUM. Once the stress period is past, adrenal activity decreases and diuresis begins. At this time, usually after the second to the fifth postoperative day, daily potassium is given to prevent a deficit; potassium is not conserved by the body but lost in the urine. Electrolyte maintenance fluids may be used or potassium may be added to parenteral solutions; usually 40 mEq per liter daily is sufficient to replace normal loss. Potassium should be well diluted and the rate should not exceed 20 to 30 mEq per hour. A slower rate of administration is preferred for older patients. Usually 40 mEq is infused over an 8 hour period. The solution containing potassium should be conspicuously labeled and must never be used when positive pressure is indicated—rapid infusion may result in cardiac arrest.

Potassium is irritating to the vein and may cause a great deal of pain, especially if infused into a vein where a previous venipuncture has been performed. Slowing the rate may decrease the pain.

VITAMINS. Vitamins B complex and C are usually added to parenteral solutions if, after 2 or 3 days, the patient is unable to take fluids orally. Vitamin C is important in promoting healing in the surgical patient and vitamin B complex is helpful in aiding in carbohydrate metabolism.

PARENTERAL THERAPY FOR THE BURNED PATIENT

The body mechanisms that regulate fluid and electrolyte balance are altered when severe burns occur. The changes that take place during the first 48 hours must be recognized and dealt with. Fluid and electrolyte therapy sufficient to replace losses and maintain a status quo increase the patient's chances of survival. Awareness of these physiological changes contributes to intelligent therapy and aids in the patient's recovery.

FLUID AND ELECTROLYTE CHANGES

INTRAVASCULAR TO INTERSTITIAL FLUID SHIFT. The shift from intravascular to interstitial fluid, followed by shock, begins immediately following the burn. This fluid shift represents the water, electrolyte, and protein that are lost through the damaged capillaries, resulting in edema and a marked reduction in plasma volume. The severity of the shift depends upon the degree and extent of the burn. In an adult with a 50 percent burn, the edema may exceed the total plasma volume of the patient. Parenteral fluids must be given immediately to replace the fluid loss and combat shock.

DEHYDRATION. In the early phases of fluid shift from plasma to tissues, water and electrolyte are lost in larger quantities than the protein (protein, because of its larger molecular size, does not readily pass through the capillary walls). The osmotic pressure, increased by the higher protein concentration of the plasma, draws fluid from the undamaged tissues and generalized tissue dehydration occurs.

A much more significant fluid loss occurs as (1) exudate from the burned area, (2) water in the form of vapor at the burned area, and (3) blood lost through the damaged capillaries. These losses further contribute to dehydration and hypovolemia.

DECREASED URINARY OUTPUT. Decreased urinary output occurs when the lowered blood volume causes a diminished renal blood flow. Increased endocrine secretions further contribute to the decrease in urinary output: adrenal cortical secretions cause sodium and water absorption; ADH causes increased water reabsorption by the kidneys.

In deep burns free hemoglobin, released by destruction of red cells, may produce renal damage.

POTASSIUM EXCESS. When excessive amounts of potassium build up in the extracellular fluid, potassium excess occurs: cell destruction releases potassium and decreased renal flow obstructs normal excretion of potassium. Plasma potassium concentrations may rise to a dangerously high level. Because of the tendency of plasma potassium excess and the uncertain extent of renal impairment, administration of potassium is contraindicated.

SODIUM DEFICIT. When plasma is lost in edema and exudate, sodium, chief electrolyte of the extracellular fluid, is lost with the plasma, and sodium deficit occurs. Further loss may occur as sodium moves into the cells to replace lost potassium.

METABOLIC ACIDOSIS. Acidosis results from a loss of bicarbonate ions accompanying the loss of sodium ions as well as altered aerobic metabolized tissue destruction.

FLUID THERAPY

When moderate or severe burns occur, immediate fluid therapy is necessary to combat hypovolemic shock and prevent renal depression. An indwelling venous catheter is inserted to ensure parenteral therapy during this critical period. As the measurement of venous pressure is an important guide against overinfusion, a second catheter may be inserted for venous pressure determination.

In small burns that require parenteral therapy, solutions such as isotonic saline, Ringer's solution, or 5 percent dextrose in water or saline may be sufficient, but in severe burns a colloid is usually employed. Colloids, because of their tendency to hold fluids in the vascular compartment, are used to maintain blood volume and combat shock. Plasma, albumin, and dextran are the most common of the colloidal solutions used. Whole blood is added when indicated.

Fluid therapy consists in supplying (1) the normal daily fluid requirements and (2) additional amounts of fluid for replacement of burn losses. The amount of fluid necessary to replace burn losses is calculated in relation to the extent and severity of the burn. The "rule of nines" is the most common used to estimate the burned area. The surface area of the body is divided into areas of 9 percent or its multiples (see Table 7).

During the first 24 hours, a great deal more fluid is required to replace the marked reduction in plasma volume caused by the rapid shift of intravascular to interstitial fluid.

TABLE 7. "Rule of Nines" for Estimation of Burned Body Area

Part of Body	Percentage of Body
Head and neck	9
Anterior trunk	18
Each arm	9
Posterior trunk	18
Genitalia	1
Each leg	18

This fluid replacement increases the total body water content, secondary to the burn edema, and results in a weight gain. This gain may be as much as 10 percent of the normal body weight [4].

Caution must be taken to avoid overzealous fluid therapy. Later when fluid shifts back into the plasma excess parenteral fluid could cause overburdened circulation and pulmonary edema. If smoke and heat damage to the lungs have impaired their capacity to function, the threat of pulmonary edema is further increased. Only enough fluid to maintain blood volume and urinary output is administered.

The shift from interstitial fluid to plasma begins on the second to third day after the burn and accounts for the large reduction in parenteral fluids. An increase in the urinary output should alert the nurse to the edema mobilization taking place and the need to decrease fluid therapy.

Massachusetts General Hospital's principles of fluid replacement

Various formulas based on fluid needs for the first 24 hours have been developed to serve as a guide to fluid therapy. Such estimates are helpful in reducing the danger of overhydration or underhydration that exists during the critical period.

In the years following the fire in 1942 at the Coconut Grove (a Boston nightclub), the Massachusetts General Hospital made great strides in introducing theory and principles beneficial to burn therapy. Immediately after a burn, edema begins to develop in the involved area. The description of the nature of this fluid and protein loss into the interstitial compartment was accomplished to a great extent by Dr. Oliver Cope.

The Massachusetts General Hospital and the Shriners Burns Institute employ their own formula and principles of fluid replacement based on the belief that "the normal fluid environment of the tissues is the optimal one and there is no good evidence that healing or survival is improved by any variations" [4]. Consequently the fluid program is based upon an attempt to replace fluid loss with similar fluid.

In severe burns a large amount of water is lost through the damaged skin and this must be replaced. The fluid lost in edema contains about 4.5 gm of protein per 100 ml, which is less protein than the 6 to 7 gm normally present in plasma [4]. The concentration of electrolytes generally remains about the same. The blood bank plasma that is available usually has a protein content slightly higher (between 4.5 and 5 gm per 100 ml) than the burn edema fluid and, in some cases, a sodium content somewhat lower [4]. Therefore plasma is used either alone or with small amounts of saline to make an isotonic solution with a protein content of about 4.5 gm per 100 ml.

Because of the potential risk of serum hepatitis to the patient infused with pooled plasma, the amount of available plasma is limited; only single donor plasma is used. Other colloids such as albumin and dextran may be substituted. Frequently normal human albumin prepared in a 5 percent solution is used. However, if other protein fractions, such as gamma globulin, are indicated they must be given as a supplement.

Whole blood is used cautiously during the first 48 hours in the belief that only proved blood losses should be replaced. A decreased red blood cell volume is not usually apparent until 48 hours after the burn when the red cells damaged by the heat become increasingly more fragile and hemolyze. Slow administration of blood during the critical period may delay the urgent need for the more vitally needed fluid.

Fluid requirements based on Massachusetts General Hospital's replacement principles

The following schedule of fluid replacement is followed at Massachusetts General Hospital in accord with the principles [4] just elucidated:

first 24 hours

Normal fluid requirements

2000 ml of nonelectrolyte solution (5 percent dextrose in water)

Replacement of burn loss

Plasma with approximately 5 gm protein/100 ml, amount determined by degree of burn (125 ml plasma per percentage of body area burned)

Saline amount determined by degree of burn (15 ml saline per percentage of body area burned)

One half of the first 24-hour total amount infused in first 8 hours and the rest in 16 remaining hours

SECOND 24 HOURS

Normal fluid requirements

2000 ml of 5 percent dextrose in water

Replacement of burn loss

One half of the previous 24-hour requirement

Because it is believed that each patient should be treated on an individual basis, the formula gives only a rough approximation of amount of fluid that should be infused and is used only while the critical period exists. Physicians still vary in their opinions on replacement fluid. Some prefer to treat the patient clinically, relying on Ringer's lactate solution.

BROOKE ARMY HOSPITAL FORMULA

The Brooke Army Hospital formula [5] is one of the most widely used formulas.

FIRST 24 HOURS

Normal fluid requirements

2000 ml of nonelectrolyte solution (5 percent dextrose in water)

Replacement of burn loss

Colloid and electrolyte solution in ratio of 1 to 3 with amount of replacement fluid equaling 2 ml × kg body weight × percentage of body area burned

One half of this total amount infused in first 8 hours and the rest in 16 remaining hours

SECOND 24 HOURS

Normal fluid requirements

2000 ml of 5 percent dextrose in water

Replacement of burn loss

One half the amount of colloid and electrolyte solution of the first 24 hours

The Evans formula is probably considered one of the best known. It is much the same as the Brooke formula with the exception that equal proportions of colloid and electrolyte solutions are used. This ratio was originally based on the belief that the fluid lost in edema contained 50 percent plasma.

Parenteral therapy after critical phase

After 48 hours, when the edema remobilization period is reached, colloids are stopped and parenteral fluids are curtailed or discontinued to prevent expanded fluid volume with pulmonary edema. The amount of fluid then administered parenterally depends upon the patient's ability to take fluid orally.

During the convalescent phase care is taken to provide necessary electrolytes to prevent or correct a deficit of sodium, potassium, and calcium.

Fluid therapy for the burned child

Fluid replacement for the burned child is essentially the same as for the adult with the exception of the calculation of the percentage of surface area involved. See Table 8 for estimations of these percentages.

The tentative plan of fluid therapy for the burned child is 90 ml of plasma and 10 ml of saline for each percentage of burned area times the body surface area in square meters [4]. Greater accuracy in fluid administration is necessary than for the adult, as the child is more sensitive to minor errors, developing pulmonary edema and shock more quickly.

TABLE 8. Chart for Estimating Burned Area in Children

Part of Body	Percentage of Body	
	0–4 yr	4–10 yr
Head	16	12
Neck	2	2
Trunk (whole)	32	32
Each arm	8	9
Each leg	16	18

SOURCE: Abbott Laboratories [1].

DIABETIC ACIDOSIS

Diabetic acidosis is an endocrine disorder causing complex fluid and electrolyte disturbances. It occurs when a lack of insulin prevents the metabolism of glucose, and essential calories are provided by the catabolism of fat and protein. Acidosis results from the accumulation of acid by-products. Knowledge of the physiological changes in diabetic acidosis aids the nurse in early detection of imbalances and in an understanding of the treatment involved.

Physiological changes

Lack of insulin prevents cellular metabolism of glucose and its conversion into glycogen. Glucose accumulates in the blood stream (*hyperglycemia*). When the blood sugar rises above 180 mg per 100 ml, glucose spills over into the urine (*glycosuria*). The kidneys require 10 to 20 ml of water to excrete 1 gm of glucose; water excretion increases (*polyuria*).

The body's fat and protein are utilized to provide necessary calories for energy. Ketone bodies, metabolic by-products, reduce plasma bicarbonate, and acidosis occurs.

Fluid and electrolyte disturbances

DEHYDRATION. Dehydration results from excessive fluid and electrolyte losses. Cellular fluid deficit occurs when water is drawn from the cells by the hyperosmolality of the blood.

Extracellular deficit occurs when (1) glycosuria increases the urinary output, (2) ketone bodies increase the load on the kidneys and the water to excrete them, (3) vomiting causes loss of fluid and electrolytes, (4) oral intake is reduced because of the patient's condition, and (5) hyperventilation is induced by the acidic state.

DECREASED KIDNEY FUNCTION. Dehydration lowers the blood volume, decreasing renal blood flow, and the kidneys produce less of the ammonia needed to maintain acid–base balance. Severe dehydration may lower the blood volume enough to cause circulatory shock and oliguria.

KETOSIS. Ketosis is the excessive production of ketone bodies in the blood stream. Electrolytes and ketone bodies, retained in high serum concentration, increase the acidosis; the increase in the number of H^+, from the retention of ketone bodies, may drop the blood pH to as low as 6.9. The bicarbonate anions decrease to compensate for the increase in ketone anions and may drop the bicarbonate level as low as 5 mEq per liter [8].

ELECTROLYTE CHANGES. Cellular potassium deficit occurs when cells, unable to metabolize glucose, break down and release potassium into the serum. Normal or high serum potassium concentration may exist in spite of a body deficit (98 percent of the body's potassium is contained in the cells). Increase in the concentration of serum potassium is the result of the large amounts of potassium released from the cells plus the increased retention of potassium due to impaired kidney function. In severe diabetic acidosis, serious sodium and chloride deficits may occur when these electrolytes are lost through diuresis, vomiting, and gastric dilatation.

Signs and symptoms of diabetic acidosis

The nurse should be familiar with the signs and symptoms that characterize diabetic acidosis. By recognizing impending diabetic acidosis, early treatment may be initiated and complications prevented.

1. *Hyperglycemia* occurs when a lack of insulin prevents glucose metabolism; glucose accumulates in the blood stream.
2. *Glycosuria* occurs when the accumulation of glucose exceeds the renal tolerance and spills over into the urine.
3. *Polyuria.* Osmotic diuresis occurs when the heavy load of nonmetabolized glucose and the metabolic end products increase the osmolality of the blood, and the increased renal solute load requires more fluid for excretion.
4. *Thirst* is prompted by cellular dehydration due to the osmotic effect produced by hyperglycemia.
5. *Weakness, tiredness* comes from the inability of the body to utilize glucose and from a potassium deficit.
6. *Flushed face* results from the acid condition.
7. *Rapid deep breathing* is the body's defense against acidosis; expiration of large amounts of CO_2 reduce carbonic acid and increase the pH of the blood.
8. *Acetone breath* results from an increased accumulation of acetone bodies.
9. *Nausea, vomiting* are caused by distention due to atony of gastric muscles.
10. *Weight loss* accompanies an excess loss of fluid (1 liter of body water equals 2.2 pounds or 1 kg body weight) and a lack of glucose metabolism.
11. *Low blood pressure* results from a severe fluid deficit.
12. *Oliguria* follows the decreased renal blood flow that results from a severe deficit in fluid volume.

PARENTERAL THERAPY

Insulin is given to metabolize the excess glucose and combat diabetic acidosis. Since absorption by the blood stream is quickest, insulin is administered intravenously. When given subcutaneously or intramuscularly, the slower rate of absorption of insulin may be further decreased by peripheral collapse in the presence of shock.

Parenteral fluids are administered to increase the blood volume and restore kidney function. Hypotonic solutions with sodium chloride (usually containing sodium lactate or bicarbonate) are employed. These provide the basic needs for water, sodium, and alkali of the acidic patient, thus hydrating him and reducing the acidosis. Solutions of glucose may be needed to prevent hypoglycemia and are sometimes used at the onset of treatment. Some physicians feel that the glucose increases the hyperglycemia, causing increased diuresis with further loss of water and electrolytes [8]. For this reason they prefer to wait 4 to 6 hours until the available glucose has been metabolized before administering glucose solutions.

Frequently isotonic solutions of sodium chloride are used to replace sodium and chloride losses and expand the blood volume.

Potassium administration is contraindicated in the early treatment of diabetic acidosis. During the later stages (10 to 24 hours after treatment) the plasma potassium level falls; improved renal function increases potassium excretion and, in anabolic states, as the glucose is converted into glycogen, a sudden shift of potassium from extracellular fluid to intracellular fluid further lowers the plasma potassium level. If the patient is hydrated, potassium should be administered when the plasma potassium concentration falls.

A severe potassium deficit may occur if symptoms are not recognized and early treatment begun. Symptoms include weak grip, irregular pulse, weak picking at the bed clothes, shallow respiration, and abdominal distention.

REFERENCES

1. Abbott Laboratories. *Fluid and Electrolytes.* North Chicago, Ill., 1960. Pp. 45–46.
2. Adriani, J. Venipuncture. *American Journal of Nursing* 62:66, 1962.

3. Burgess, R. E. Fluid and electrolytes. *American Journal of Nursing* 65:90, 1965.
4. Burke, J. F., and Constable, J. D. Systemic changes and replacement therapy in burns. *Journal of Trauma* 5:242–253, 1965.
5. Collentine, G. E., Jr. How to calculate fluids for burned patients. *American Journal of Nursing* 62:77, 1962.
6. Elman, R. Fluid balance from the nurse's point of view. *American Journal of Nursing* 49:222, 1949.
7. McGaw Laboratories. *Guide to Parenteral Fluid Therapy.* Glendale, Cal., 1963. P. 63.
8. Metheny, N. M., and Snively, W. D., Jr. *Nurses' Handbook of Fluid Balance.* Philadelphia: Lippincott, 1967. Pp. 103, 122, 147–154, 157–169, 177, 218.
9. Talbot, N. B., Sobel, E. H., McArthur, J. W., and Crawford, J. D. *Functional Endocrinology from Birth Through Adolescence.* Cambridge, Mass.: Harvard University Press, 1952.

10.

Intravenous Administration of Drugs

NOT SO LONG AGO the subcutaneous and the intramuscular routes were the preferred routes for the parenteral administration of drugs. With the success of and increase in intravenous therapy, the practice grew of including drugs in infusions. Today intravenous therapy is used extensively for drug administration.

ADVANTAGES

The venous route for drug administration offers pronounced advantages which are given below.

1. Some drugs cannot be absorbed by any other route; the large molecular size of some drugs prevents absorption by the gastrointestinal route while other drugs, unstable in the presence of gastric juices, are destroyed.
2. Certain drugs, because of their irritating properties, cause pain and trauma when given by the intramuscular or subcutaneous routes and must be given intravenously.
3. The vascular system affords a method for providing instant drug action.
4. The intravenous route offers a better control over the rate of administration of drugs; prolonged action can be provided

by administering a dilute infusion intermittently or over a prolonged period of time.

5. The vascular route affords a route of administration for the patient who cannot tolerate fluids and drugs by the gastrointestinal route.

6. Slow intravenous administration of the drug permits termination of the infusion if sensitivity occurs.

HAZARDS

In spite of the advantages offered by the venous route, there are certain hazards which are not found in other forms of drug therapy.

1. Possibility of incompatibilities when one or more drugs are added to the intravenous solution
2. Speed shock (a systemic reaction to a substance rapidly injected into the blood stream)
3. Vascular irritations and subsequent hazards
4. Rapid onset of action with inability to recall drug once it has entered the blood stream

INCOMPATIBILITIES

The number of possible drug combinations, provided by the ever-increasing production of drugs and parenteral fluids, is astronomical. With the increase in drug combinations comes an increase in potential incompatibilities. How and why incompatibilities occur and how best to avoid them are problems confronting all those involved in compounding intravenous additives. However well we know the chemical action of one group of drugs, our knowledge falls short when many groups are combined into complex compounds. The nurse, confronted with these problems, faces increased responsibility.

Many hospitals have set up pharmacy-centralized intravenous additive programs. This places the responsibility for prescription compounding with the department best qualified to assume it. The pharmacist is best able to predict or to detect incompatibilities and is alert to prescribed errors. The greater opportunity for sterility and accuracy when drugs are prepared in the pharmacy is obviously an advantage.

However, if such a pharmacy-centralized intravenous additive program is lacking, the responsibility is often left with the nurse. The pharmacist must be directly available, alerting her to possible chemical incompatibilities, communicating with various manufacturers on specific pharmaceutical problems, and providing information on certain drugs. An inservice program should be instituted, supplying an approved list of drugs for administration and acquainting the nurse with reactions, contraindications, dosage, stability, and compatibilities.

The individual who mixes and compounds intravenous drugs must be alert to the hazards of drug therapy. Since incompatibilities are a complication of prime consideration in the preparation of solutions, the nurse should have an acquaintance with the concepts involved in this hazard.

Compatibility charts are available but generally show only physical incompatibilities. Even chemical compatibility charts may be useless because of differences in the drug formation from one manufacturer to another or because of changes made by one manufacturer. The order of mixing drugs, the quantity of the drug and the solution, room temperature, and light contribute to incompatibilities not noted on the chart. Incompatibilities are not always obvious, as chemical changes may occur which do not produce a visible change.

Precipitation may occur when one or more drugs are added to parenteral solution [11]. It does not always occur at the time the solution is prepared, which increases the problem of intravenous administration. Some drugs, stable for a limited period of time, degrade and may or may not precipitate as they become less therapeutically active. If administered intravenously, solutions containing insoluble matter carry potential danger of embolism, myocardial damage, and effect on other organs such as the liver and the kidneys.

Chemical interactions

The most common incompatibilities are the result of certain chemical reactions [11].

1. *Hydrolysis* is the process in which water absorption causes decomposition of a compound. In preparing solutions of salt, the nurse should understand that certain salts, when placed in water, hydrolyze, forming a very strong acid and a weak base, or a weak acid and a strong base. Since pH is a significant factor in the solubility of drugs, the increased acidity or alkalinity from hydrolysis of a salt may result in an incompatibility if another drug is added.

Example of hydrolysis: The acid salt, sodium bicarbonate, when placed in water hydrolyzes to form a strong alkali (sodium hydroxide) and a weak and unstable acid (carbonic acid). Many organic acids are known as weak acids since they ionize only slightly [8].

2. *Reduction* is the process whereby one or more atoms gain electrons at the expense of some other part of the system [5].

3. *Oxidation* is the corresponding loss of electrons occurring when reduction takes place. Antioxidants are often used as a preservative to prevent oxidation of a compound [5].

4. *Double decomposition* is the chemical reaction in which ions of two compounds change places and two new compounds are thus formed [8]. A great many salts act by double decomposition to form other salts and probably represent the largest number of incompatibilities.

Example: Calcium chloride is incompatible with sodium bicarbonate; the double decomposition results in the formation of the insoluble salt calcium carbonate.

Classification of incompatibilities

Incompatibilities may be divided into three categories:

1. *Therapeutic.* An undesirable reaction resulting from over-

lapping effects of two drugs given together or close together.

2. *Physical.* According to Endicott [13], "The term 'physical incompatibility' is somewhat misleading but has come to be accepted as a physical or chemical interaction between two or more ingredients which leads to a visible change in the mixture which can be readily observed." A visible change may not occur when many chemical reactions take place. The physical change may be:
   a) Gas formation, such as occurs when carbonates are placed in acid. (Sodium bicarbonate in acid forms carbon dioxide gas.)
   b) Color change, such as occurs when riboflavin in vitamin B complex and methylene blue form a green color.
   c) Precipitation, occurring when compounds are insoluble. (Acid salts in alkali cause free base to precipitate; base salts in acid cause free acid to precipitate.) [11].
3. *Chemical.* A chemical change is here classified as a change in drug compounds which is not readily observed. Since it may go undetected it has a greater capacity for causing biological effects.

pH AND ITS ROLE IN STABILITY OF DRUGS

Since pH plays an important role in the solubility of drugs it may be well to define it. pH is the symbol for the degree of concentration of hydrogen ions or the acidity of the solution. The weight of H ions in 1 liter of pure water is 0.0000001 gm, which is numerically equal to 10^{-7}. For convenience, the negative logarithm 7 is used. Since it is at this concentration that the hydrogen ions balance the hydroxyl ions, a pH of 7 is neutral. Each unit decrease in pH represents a tenfold increase in H ions [8].

It appears likely that the largest number of incompatibilities may be produced by changes in pH [10]. Precipitation occurs when a compound is insoluble in solution. The degree of solubility often varies with the pH. A drastic change in the pH of a drug when added to an intravenous solution suggests an incompatibility or a decrease in stability. Solutions of a high pH appear to be incompatible with solutions of a low pH and may form insoluble free acids or free bases. A chart denoting the pH of certain drugs and certain solutions to be used as a vehicle is helpful in warning of potential incompatibilities.

FACTORS AFFECTING STABILITY OR pH. Many factors may affect the stability or pH of drugs:

1. *Parenteral solutions.* Some commonly prescribed drugs precipitate when added to intravenous solutions. Over ninety different infusion solutions, along with their pH, are listed by one company alone. Differences in the physical and chemical properties of each of these solutions may affect the stability of any drug introduced. A compound, soluble in one solution, may precipitate in another. Sodium ampicillin deteriorates in acid solutions. This drug, when added to isotonic sodium chloride at a concentration of 30 mg per milliliter, loses less than 10 percent activity in 8 hours. However, when added to 5 percent dextrose in water, usually a more acid solution, its stability is reduced to a 4-hour period.

Another factor affecting the stability of drugs is the broad pH range (3.5 to 6.5) of dextrose solutions allowed by the USP. "A drug may be stable in one bottle of dextrose 5 percent in water and not in another" [2].

2. *Additional drugs.* One drug may be compatible in a solution, but a second additive may alter the established pH to such an extent as to make the drugs unstable [9].

3. *Buffering agents in drugs.* An important consideration in the stability of drugs is the presence of buffers or antioxidants which may cause two drugs, however compatible, to precipitate. For example, ascorbic acid, the buffering component of tetracycline, lowers the pH of the product and therefore may accelerate the decomposition of a drug susceptible to an acid environment.

4. *Preservatives in the diluent.* Sterile diluents for reconstitution of drugs are available with or without a bacteriostatic agent. The bacteriostatic agents usually consist of parabens or phenol preservatives. Certain drugs, including nitrofurantoin, amphotericin B, and erythromycin, are incompatible with these preservatives and should be reconstituted with sterile water for injection.

5. *Degree of dilution.* Solubility often varies with the volume of solution in which a drug is introduced. For example, tetracycline HCl, mixed in a small volume of fluid, maintains its pH range over 24 hours. However, when added to a large volume (1 liter), it degrades after 12 hours, becoming less therapeutically active.

6. *Period of time solution stands.* Decomposition of substances in solution is proportional to the length of time they stand. For example, dextrose solutions are unstable when maintained in a neutral or basic environment. Therefore it is recommended that when bicarbonate is to be added to dextrose solutions, it be added immediately prior to use [6].

7. *Order of mixing.* The order in which drugs are added to infusions often determines their compatibility.

8. *Light.* Light may provide energy for chemical reactions to occur. Therefore certain drugs, such as amphotericin B and nitrofurantoin, once diluted must be protected from light [9].

9. *Room temperature.* Heat also provides energy for reactions. After reconstitution or initial dilution, refrigeration prolongs the stability of many drugs.

VASCULAR IRRITATION

The hazards of intravenous therapy can be reduced by adequate precautions (see Chapter 7).

Vascular irritation is a significant hazard of drugs intravenously administered. Any irritation that inflames and roughens the endothelial cells of the venous wall allows platelets to adhere; a thrombus is formed. Thrombophlebitis is the result of the sterile inflammation. When a thrombus occurs, there is always the inherent danger of embolism.

If aseptic technique is not strictly adhered to, a septic thrombophlebitis may result from bacteria introduced through the infusion needle and becoming trapped in the thrombus. This is much more serious, as it carries with it the potential dangers of septicemia and acute bacterial endocarditis.

PREVENTIVE MEASURES

The following adequate precautions must be observed to diminish the potential hazards of vascular irritation:

1. Veins with ample blood volume should be selected when infusing hypertonic solutions or solutions containing irritating compounds.
2. The needle should be appreciably smaller than the lumen of the vein. A large needle may occlude the lumen, obstructing the flow of blood; the solution then flows undiluted, irritating the wall of the vein.
3. The venipuncture should be performed at the distal end of the extremity to allow each successive puncture to be executed proximal to the previous. Hypertonic solutions, when allowed to flow through a traumatized vein, cause increased irritation and pain.
4. Veins in the lower extremities are prone to trauma and should be avoided.
5. Isotonic solutions should, when possible, follow hypertonic solutions to wash irritating substances from the veins.
6. The rate of infusion may contribute to the irritation. (1) In a large vein, slow administration permits greater dilution of the drug with the circulating blood. (2) In a small vein lacking ample circulating blood, a slow drip prolongs the irritation, increasing the inflammation.
7. Prolonged duration of an infusion increases the risk of phlebitis. After a 24-hour period the danger increases. Periodic inspection of the injection site to detect a developing phlebitis

is important. After 72 hours the injection site should be changed.

8. Precautions should be observed to avoid administering solutions containing particulate matter by

a) Proper reconstitution and dilution of additives
b) Inspection of parenteral fluids before administration
c) Use of freshly prepared solutions
d) Use of a set with a filter when danger of precipitation exists
e) Periodic inspection of solutions containing additives
f) Avoidance of administration of cloudy solutions unless affirmed by the manufacturer

RESPONSIBILITY OF HOSPITAL COMMITTEE

The special committee which deals with problems concerning therapeutic procedures should

1. Provide the nurse with an approved list of medications that may be added to parenteral solutions
2. Delineate the types of fluids she may administer
3. Provide an inservice program to acquaint the nurse with reactions, contraindications, dosage, and effects

PHYSICIAN'S RESPONSIBILITY

The physician writes and signs all orders for intravenous fluids and drug solutions. In each case the doctor should specify the rate of flow either as milliliters per hour or the approximate length of time of administration of the infusion.

He is responsible for administering intravenously all medications not on the list approved for nurses. This usually consists of certain types of drugs such as

1. Those which may produce a severe immediate reaction [12]. *Example:* Nitrogen mustard, iron preparations, and

other drugs in which the possibility of anaphylaxis is of prime concern.

2. Those whose dose is dependent upon the response of the patient and which are to be injected directly into the vein [12]. *Example:* Epinephrine—dilution permits slow infusion and minimizes occurrence of reactions.
3. Those whose extravasation may result in necrosis [12]. *Example:* Levarterenol bitartrate. Infiltration of this drug may lead to severe sloughing of the tissues. It increases the blood pressure by producing peripheral venous restriction, resulting in ischemia of the skin.

INTRAVENOUS NURSE'S RESPONSIBILITY

The following tasks are the responsibility of the intravenous nurse. She

1. Checks the doctor's book for all complete orders of intravenous therapy. If a doubt exists regarding the compatibility or safety of a drug, the physician or pharmacist should be consulted.
2. Compounds only the drugs on the authorized list.
3. Labels solution, indicating patient's name, drug, amount, date, time prepared, and her signature.
4. Delivers compounded, labeled solution to patient's unit, substantiating identification of patient and compounded solution. The nurse is legally responsible for all drugs and solutions that she prepares and administers.
5. Initiates the infusion and adjusts the rate of flow. No coercion should be used on rational, adult patients. If the patient refuses the infusion, the nurse should notify the physician in charge of the patient.
6. Questions patient regarding sensitivity to drugs which may cause anaphylaxis. Observes patient for a short time following initial administration of such drugs. If a question of sensitivity exists, the drug should be administered by the physician.

RESPONSIBILITY OF THE ATTENDING NURSE

The nurse in attendance is responsible for maintaining the infusion. Through periodic inspection she

1. Regulates and maintains the prescribed rate of flow.
2. Observes the injection site for any developing complications before serious damage occurs. If phlebitis or infiltration occurs, she removes the needle.
3. Hangs consecutive bottles of intravenous fluid, inspecting compounded solutions for precipitation.
4. Discontinues intravenous therapy, taking care to prevent hematomas from occurring by applying firm pressure over puncture site for at least 2 minutes, or longer if necessary.

NURSES' INTRAVENOUS ADDITIVE STATION

An especially equipped additive unit creates an environment of safety for the preparation of parenteral admixtures. This unit should provide the following:

1. *Isolated clean area.* Medications should be prepared in an area that permits complete concentration, since distraction increases the potential risk of human error.

As traffic generates airborne contamination, an isolated area provides a better opportunity for sterility. The air in the typical hospital includes tiny contaminating particles, such as dust, lint, medication, and spores, in constant motion. These particles provide lodgment on which airborne bacteria thrive. The increased activity of bedmaking, sweeping, and other functions increases the degree of airborne particles and provides an environment which interferes with aseptic technique and may contribute to contamination [1].

2. *Laminar flow hood.* Some additive stations are equipped with a laminar flow unit to provide a clean work area where aseptic techniques can be performed. The concept of such a unit was evolved in 1961 and defined by Federal Standard 209a

[3] as "air flow in which the entire body of air within a confined area moves with uniform velocity along parallel flow lines, with a minimum of eddies." These units, available in small bench models, play an important role in delineating the hazard of airborne contamination of intravenous solutions.

3. *Proper illumination.* Adequate light permits visualization of particulate matter. Black and white backgrounds aid in the visual detection of these foreign substances. Laminar flow units provide illumination by fluorescent light [4].

4. *Supplies.* A complete stock of equipment should be available, including

a) Parenteral solutions and administration sets
b) Syringes and needles
c) Commonly used intravenous additives
d) Diluents
  (1) Sterile bacteriostatic water injection USP
  (2) Sterile water injection USP
  (3) Normal saline injection USP
e) Container for the proper disposal of needles and syringes

5. A list of drugs and drug combinations approved for intravenous administration by nurses should be posted.

PREPARATION OF INTRAVENOUS SOLUTIONS AND ADDITIVES

Extreme care in the preparation of solutions diminishes the risks associated with intravenous therapy.

1. *Aseptic technique is imperative.* Pyrogenic contamination of drug products and parenteral solutions must be avoided.

2. *Proper dilution of lyophilized drugs is essential.* Two special cautions to assure complete solubility in the reconstitution of drugs must be observed: (1) The specific diluent recommended by the manufacturer should be used. (2) The drug should be initially diluted in the volume recommended.

3. *Introduction of extraneous particles into parenteral solu-*

tions must be avoided. Fragments of rubber stoppers are frequently cut out by the needles used and accidentally injected into solutions [7]. Large bore (15-gauge) needles are practical for use in the nurses' station and appear to provide less disadvantage than the smaller needles. (1) Smaller needles may encourage particles which may be difficult to see on inspection. (2) The small particles may be of a size capable of passing through the indwelling needle.

A solution which upon inspection contains fragments of rubber must be discarded or filtered. There is a set available which provides filtration to 0.45 microns.

Procedure in compounding and administering parenteral solutions

The following steps should be carried out in the preparation of solutions for infusion:

1. Substantiate drug orders with the drug product and the parenteral solution.
2. Inspect solution for extraneous particles.
3. Check drug product for
   a) Expiration date: Outdated drugs should not be used, as loss of potency or stability may have occurred.
   b) Method of administration: (1) Intramuscular preparations are not usually used for intravenous administration; they may contain certain components such as anesthetics or preservatives not meant for administration by vascular route. (2) Some are packaged in multiple dose vials which may contribute to contamination. (3) The dosage by intramuscular route may not coincide with that for intravenous use.
4. With an accepted antiseptic, clean rubber injection site of both the drug product and the diluent.
5. Use sterile syringe and needle.
6. Reconstitute according to manufacturer's recommendation.

TABLE 9. Solubility of Medications in Commonly Used Intravenous Fluids

DRUG	pH Range→ ↓	Dextrose 5% or 10% in Water 3.5-6.5	Sodium Chloride 0.9% 5.0-6.0	Lactated Ringer's 6.0-7.5	REMARKS AND "PRODUCT MAY ALSO CONTAIN"
Aminophylline	8.5-8.9	S	S	S	Ethylenediamine
Ammonium Chloride	4.0-6.0	S	S	S	
Amphotericin B	7.0	S*	I	I	Sodium phosphates, sodium desoxycholate
Arginine Glutamate	5.8	S	S	S	Glutamic acid, sodium bisulfite
Ascorbic Acid	5.5-7.0	S	S	S	As sodium ascorbate. Sodium sulfite, sodium bisulfite
Calcium Chloride	6.5-8.5	S	S	S	
Calcium Disodium Edetate	6.5-8.0	S	S	–	
Calcium Gluceptate	6.2	S	S	S	Monothioglycerol
Cephaloridine	5.2	S	S	–	
Corticotropin	3.0-7.0	S	S	S	Hydrolyzed gelatin
Diazepam	6.5	–	–	–	Benzyl alcohol, sodium benzoate, benzoic acid, propylene glycol, ethyl alcohol
Epinephrine HCl	2.5-5.0	S	S	S	
Erythromycin Gluceptate	6.0-8.0	S	S	S	Initial diluent should be water without preservative
Fibrinolysin	8.0-8.1	S	–	–	Glycine
Glucagon HCl	2.0	S	S	–	Glycerin, phenol
Insulin	2.5-3.5	S	S	–	
Isoproterenol HCl	3.3-5.0	S	S	S	Lactate ion, sodium bisulfite
Lincomycin HCl	3.0-5.5	S	S	S	Benzyl alcohol
Magnesium Sulfate	6.0-7.0	S	S	S	
Mannitol	6.4-6.8	S	S	–	
Menadione Sodium Bisulfite	2.0-4.0	S	S	S	Sodium bisulfite
Metaraminol Bitartrate	3.5-4.5	S	S	–	Methylparaben, propylparaben, sodium bisulfite
Methoxamine HCl	3.0-5.0	S	S	–	Citric acid, sodium citrate, potassium metabisulfite, disodium versenate, calcium chloride, methylparaben
Methyldopate HCl	3.0-6.0	S	–	–	Disodium edetate, monothioglycerol, sodium bisulfite, citric acid, parabens
Methylene Blue	3.0-4.5	S	S	S	
Oxytocin	2.5-4.5	S	S	S	Acetic acid, sodium acetate, chlorobutanol, alcohol

Phytonadione	5.0-7.0	S	S	–	Benzyl alcohol, polyoxyethylated fatty acid derivative, dextrose
Polymyxin B Sulfate	5.0-7.5	S	S	–	
Potassium Chloride	7.2	S	S	S	
Potassium Penicillin, Buffered	5.0-7.5	S	S	S	Citrates, parabens
Procainamide HCl	4.0-6.0	S	S	–	Benzyl alcohol, sodium bisulfite
Sodium Amobarbital	9.6-10.4	S[1]	S[1]	S[1]	
Sodium Ampicillin	8.5-9.5	S[2]	S[3]	–	
Sodium Bicarbonate	7.5-8.5	S	S	S	
Sodium Cephalothin	5.2	S	S	S	
Sodium Chloramphenicol-Succinate	6.4-7.0	S	S	S	
Sodium Chloride	4.5-7.0	S	S	S	
Sodium Dexamethsone Phosphate	7.5-10.5	S	S	–	Sodium citrate, methylparaben, propylparaben, sodium bisulfite, creatinine
Sodium Edetate	7.2	S	S	S	
Sodium Heparin	6.0-7.5	S	S	S	Benzyl alcohol, phenol, parabens
Sodium Hydrocortisone Phosphate	7.0-8.0	S	S	S	Phenol, sodium citrate, sodium bisulfite
Sodium Hydrocortisone-Succinate	7.0-8.0	S	S	S	Phosphates, parabens, sodium biphosphate, sodium phosphate, chlorobutanol
Sodium Menadiol Diphosphate	7.5-8.5	S	S	S	
Sodium Methicillin, Buffered	7.0-8.0	S	S	S	Sodium citrate, parabens
Sodium Methylprednisolone-Succinate	7.0-8.0	S	S	–	Phosphates, parabens
Sodium Nafcillin	6.0-6.5	I	S	S	
Sodium Novobiocin	7.5-8.5	I	S	S	Niacinamide, N-N-dimethylacetamide, benzyl alcohol
Sodium Oxacillin	6.0-8.5	S	S	–	Dibasic sodium phosphate, parabens
Sodium Pentobarbital	10.0-10.5	S[4]	S[4]	S[4]	Alcohol, propylene glycol
Sodium Phenobarbital	8.5-10.0	S[4]	S[4]	S[4]	
Sodium Prednisolone Phosphate	6.0-7.0	S	S	S	Sodium bisulfite
Sodium Secobarbital	9.7-10.5	S[4]	S[4]	S[4]	Polyethylene glycol, phenol
Sulfisoxazole Diolamine	7.3-7.8	S	S	S	Sodium metabisulfite
Tetracycline HCl	1.8-2.8	S[5]	S[5]	S[5]	Contains 2.5-3 Gms. ascorbic acid/1 Gm. tetracycline HCl
Urea	7.2	S	S	–	Citric acid
Vancomycin HCl	5.8	S	S	–	
Vitamin B Complex with C	4.0-5.1	S	S	S	Phenol, benzyl alcohol

S = Soluble
I = Incompatible
* At pH above 4.2.
** Not to be used in dextrose 10% in water.
[1] Requires at least 1.5 ml to dissolve each mg of amobarbital.
[2] Use within 4 hours.
[3] Use within 8 hours.
[4] Requires at least 1 ml to dissolve each mg of pentobarbital, phenobarbital, and secobarbital, respectively.
[5] Use within 12 hours.

7. Check diluted drug for complete solubility before adding to parenteral solution.
8. After adding to solution, invert solution bottle to mix the additive completely.
9. Clearly and properly label solution bottle:
   a) Name of patient
   b) Drug and dosage
   c) Date and time
   d) Signature
10. As added caution to prevent errors, recheck label with used drug ampules before discarding ampules.
11. Inspect solution; if necessary, use an administration set with a filter.
12. Deliver parenteral solutions to patient's unit; substantiate identity of patient with solution prepared.
13. Perform venipuncture (see Chapter 4).
14. Observe patient for a few minutes following the initial intravenous administration of any drug that may cause anaphylaxis.
15. Use added caution in administering drugs, the fast action of which could produce untoward reactions:
    a) Controlled volume set
    b) Micro drip
    c) Double clamp

General safety rules for preparation and intravenous administration of drugs by nurses

The following safety rules should be adhered to at all times:

1. Nurses will, upon written order, prepare and administer only those solutions, medications, and combinations of drugs approved in writing by the Pharmacy and Therapeutics Committee.

2. No intravenous infusion should be given that is cloudy or contains a precipitate.

3. All intravenous infusions must be used or discarded within 24 hours of the time the container is opened.

4. Any question regarding chemical compatibility or the relative safety of any drug added to an intravenous infusion should be directed to the Director of the Pharmacy.

Table 9 was prepared by John Webb, Director of the Pharmacy at Massachusetts General Hospital. It lists authorized drugs along with their pH and preservatives.

REFERENCES

1. Abbott Laboratories. *The Abbott Clean Air Center.* North Chicago, Ill., 1969.
2. Edward, M. pH—an important factor in the compatibility of additives in intravenous therapy. *American Journal of Hospital Pharmacy* 24:442, 1967.
3. Clean Room and Work Station Requirements: Controlled Environment (Federal Standard 209a). Washington, D.C.: General Services Administration, 1963.
4. Davies, W. L., and Lamy, P. P. Laminar flow. *Lippincott's Hospital Pharmacy* 3:3, 1968.
5. Degering, E. F. *Organic Chemistry* (6th ed.). New York: Barnes & Noble, 1961. P. 331.
6. Fonkalsrud, E. W., Pederson, B. M., et al. Reduction of infusion thrombophlebitis with buffered glucose solutions. *Surgery* 63:280, 1968.
7. Ho, H. F. Particulate matter in parenteral solutions. *Drug Intelligence* 1:7–25, 1967.
8. Luros, G. O., and Oram, F. *Essentials of Chemistry* (7th ed.). Philadelphia: Lippincott, 1966. Pp. 32, 74.
9. Pelissier, N. A., and Burgee, S. L. Guide to incompatibilities. *Lippincott's Hospital Pharmacy* 3:15, 1968.
10. Provost, G. E. Prescription compounding by nurses in hospitals. *American Journal of Hospital Pharmacy* 23:595, 1966.
11. Webb, J. W. A pH pattern of I.V. additives. *American Journal of Hospital Pharmacy* 26:31–35, 1969.
12. Williams, J. T., and Moravec, D. F. *Intravenous Therapy.* Hammond, Ind.: Clissold Publishing, 1967. P. 53.
13. Endicott, C. J. Workshop on Parenteral Incompatibilities. Silver Spring, Md., June 1966. *American Journal of Hospital Pharmacy* 23:599, 1966.

11.
Venous Pressure

THE MANAGEMENT OF HYPOTENSION continues to be one of the most urgent problems facing the surgeon. The parameters used in evaluating a patient in shock consist of the following [2]:

1. Blood pressure
2. Rate and quality of pulse
3. Skin temperature and color
4. Urinary output
5. Peripheral venous filling
6. Blood pH

BLOOD VOLUME DETERMINATION

New methods are increasingly available to assist in diagnosis and treatment. Of these, blood volume determination plays an important role. Maintenance of an optimal blood volume is essential for survival. Prolonged hypovolemia may cause poor tissue perfusion with the inherent risk of renal and myocardial complication; hypovolemia, uncorrected, can eventually lead to shock and death [8]. Blood volume is not necessarily reflected by the blood pressure. In cardiogenic shock the blood volume is increased and the blood pressure is low. In septic shock, hypotension accompanies a normal blood volume.

Various methods have been employed to detect change in a patient's blood volume: hematocrit, change in patient's weight, and blood volume computations before and after surgery. Blood volume determinations are an important guide during

1. *Surgery,* when the risk exists of overloading an anesthetized, traumatized patient who is continually losing blood
2. *Shock,* when origin is unknown
3. *Massive fluid replacement* in open heart surgery and in critical cases, such as the severely burned, where circulatory overload is a hazard
4. *Anuria* or *oliguria,* when questionable cause is dehydration

The Volemetron,* using radioactive isotopes, has proved extremely valuable in computing accurate blood volume determinations. Some disadvantages accompany this process: (1) the time involved, (2) the limited number that can be performed on one patient, (3) the determination quickly becomes obsolete with change produced by therapy, and (4) the expensive equipment and personnel that are needed.

VENOUS PRESSURE DETERMINATION

Venous pressure determination has overcome the disadvantages associated with the Volemetron. It requires no laboratory personnel, no expensive equipment, is simple in technique, and once set up may be monitored quickly and as often as required.

Venous pressure may be measured centrally or peripherally. *Central venous pressure* denotes the pressure in the right atrium of the venous blood as it returns from all parts of the body. The pressure varies among individuals, usually ranging between 5 and 12 cm of water (50 to 120 mm of water), but a low of 2 to 3 cm may be normal for some patients [2, 5]. The normal range has little significance since the true value lies in the change or lack of change following attempts to alter the blood volume or to improve cardiac action [2]. Since central venous pressure

* Ames Atomium Co., Elkhart, Ind.; division of Miles Laboratories, Inc.

relates to a fully sufficient circulation, it assesses both the blood volume and the ability of the heart to tolerate an increased volume, thereby providing a valuable guide for fluid administration.

Peripheral venous pressure is the pressure of the blood on the walls of the peripheral veins; to a certain extent it reflects the central venous pressure [4]. However, monitoring peripherally is less reliable: Accuracy can be affected by acute flexion of the extremity containing the catheter; thrombophlebitis or venous constriction by tumor can produce marked local elevations; poor circulation in a cold extremity may reflect only the local venous blood return, and sudden loss of blood may occur before compensatory vasoconstriction has time to take place. When accuracy is of utmost importance, caval position of the catheter is desirable.

Since central venous pressure relates to an adequate circulatory blood volume it is dependent on [3, 8]:

1. Volume of blood
2. Status of the myocardium (heart muscle)
3. Tone of blood vessels

Circulatory failure may result from deficiency in any one or combination of these essential factors.

BLOOD VOLUME. Changes in blood volume alter the tone of the blood vessels and the ability of the heart to circulate the blood. A reduced blood volume results in less pressure at the right atrium, indicated by a drop in central venous pressure; an increased blood volume produces more pressure at the atrium with a rise in central venous pressure [4].

In managing an inadequate circulation, a normal blood volume is first established. If the inadequate circulation is due to deficiency in the blood volume, manipulation is made by administering expanders; or in case of increased volume, phlebotomy.

If the circulation still remains insufficient, it becomes necessary to look at the remaining two essential components—status of the myocardium and tone of the blood vessels.

STATUS OF THE MYOCARDIUM. The status of the myocardium may be affected by disease, drugs, fluids, or anesthesia. Because the central venous pressure assesses the capacity of the myocardium as well as the blood volume, it is invaluable in monitoring the effects of anesthesia and surgery on elderly patients with arteriosclerosis or patients with myocardial insufficiency. The central venous pressure rises if the heart muscle is impaired—the pressure of the volume of blood at the heart increases because the heart muscle is no longer able to pump an adequate flow of blood out of the right atrium [4]. An elevated central venous pressure of 15 to 20 cm suggests cardiac failure [8]. This is one of the commonest causes of an elevated central venous pressure in shock.

Drugs or chemicals are administered to improve myocardial response, thus increasing cardiac output and lowering the central venous pressure.

Temporary impairment of the myocardium may be due to electrolyte imbalance and cause an early rise in central venous pressure—not above the normal range. Acidosis affects the myocardial response; if due to pulmonary insufficiency, correction is made by increasing the excretion of CO_2 [8].

TONE OF THE BLOOD VESSELS. The third essential component, the tone of the blood vessels, is dependent upon the arterial pressure and upon external and internal pressures on the veins. The arterial pressure arises from the contractile force of the left ventricle and is transmitted through the capillaries to the veins.

The external pressures upon the vein result from (1) the muscular and fascial pumping action in the extremities, (2) the intra-abdominal pressure from straining and distention, and (3) the intrathoracic pressure due to contraction of the diaphragm and chest wall. Central venous pressure of patients on positive pressure respirators is usually increased by 4 cm, while patients on negative pressure show a central venous pressure that is lower [5].

The internal pressure on the veins is due to blood volume, myocardial response, and sympathomimetic amines (epinephrine, norepinephrine). Vasopressors, by stimulating contraction of the venous wall, decrease the capacity of the venous system and improve vascular tone.

CENTRAL VENOUS PRESSURE MONITORING

Central venous pressure monitoring (see Figure 24) is achieved by attaching an intravenous set to a three-way stopcock and to an extension tube with a radiopaque catheter of approximately 24 inches. A vertical length of infusion tubing that serves as the manometer is connected to the stopcock and attached to the intravenous stand against a marked centimeter tape. Central venous pressure sets are available with disposable water manometers, graduated in units. The zero mark on the tape is adjusted to the level of the patient's right atrium. The pressure is measured at either the superior vena cava by introducing the catheter via antecubital, jugular, or subclavian vein, or at the inferior vena cava via the femoral vein.

The superior vena cava is most commonly used. Complications have been associated with inferior vena caval catheters, as reported by Bansmer et al. [1] showing 46 percent in 24 cases. In each case, with one exception, the catheter had been in place over 4 days. Use of the femoral vein and the long duration of time the catheter is in the vein enhance the risk of thrombotic complications. A second disadvantage is the fact that abdominal distention interferes with monitoring an accurate right atrial pressure.

Equipment

The following equipment is needed for monitoring venous pressure:

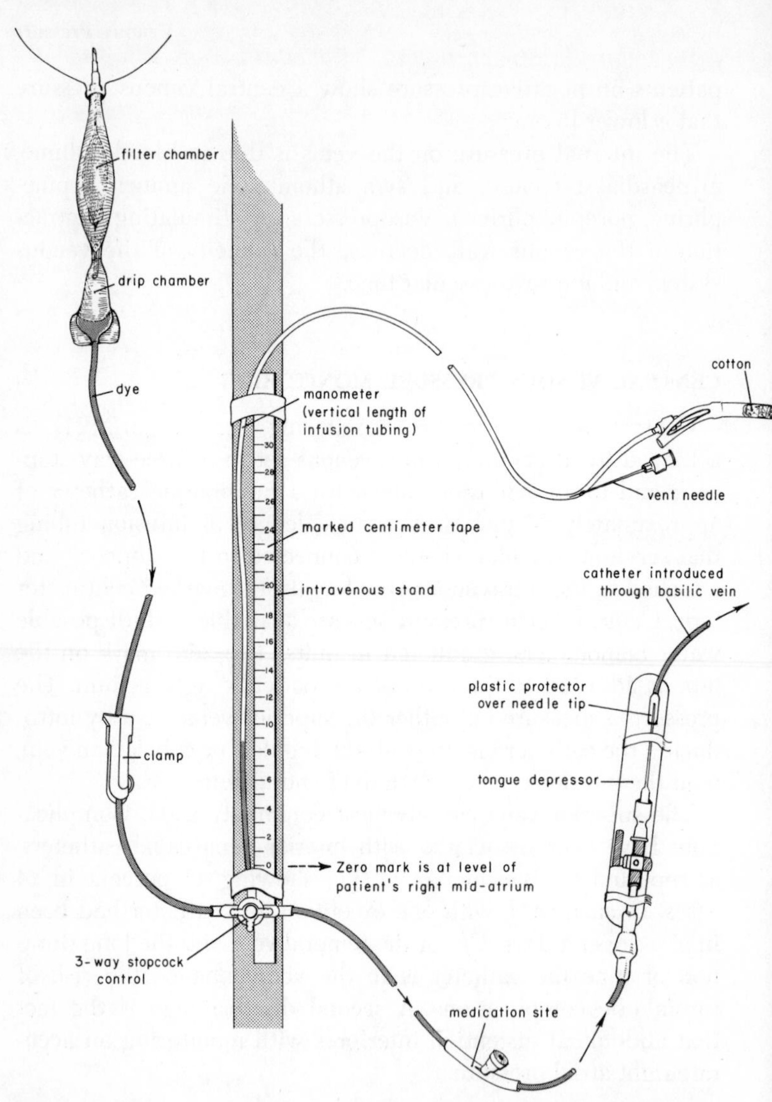

FIG. 24. Equipment for monitoring central venous pressure. Zero mark on the tape is level with the right atrium. Needle inserted into terminal end of extension tube ensures a patent vent should the cotton become wet. Notice precautions taken to prevent cutting edge of the needle from severing catheter: the bevel shield is in place and the tongue depressor provides added protection.

Intravenous Equipment	PLUS	*Venous Pressure Equipment*
Intravenous set		Local anesthetic (usually 1% procaine)
Intravenous stand		Central venous pressure set
Armboard		Catheter approximately 24 inches in length
Solution as ordered		Dye (methylene blue) if ordered
Tourniquet		Heparin 1:1000 if ordered
Antiseptic		Antibiotic ointment
Adhesive tape		Venous pressure level

PROCEDURE

Monitoring the central venous pressure is carried out as follows:

1. Explain procedure to patient.

2. Prepare solution bottles.

   Add dye (methylene blue) or vitamin B complex, if ordered.
   Facilitates reading of the manometer.

   Add heparin if ordered.
   Reduces thrombi formation and provides catheter patency.

3. Prepare equipment.

   Close three-way stopcock.

   Squeeze and hold filter chamber and insert into solution bottle.

   Completely fill filter chamber.

   Fill drip chamber one quarter full.
   Prefilling chambers prevents air bubbles from entering the manometer arm.

Tape centimeter strip onto intravenous stand with zero point adjusted to the mid-atrial level.

Patient should be in a supine position with the bed flat.

Use venous pressure level for accuracy.

Mid-atrial level is at a point approximately equidistant from the sternum and back.

Tape stopcock to pole at a level below patient's right atrium.

Do not tape directly on the stopcock (see Figure 19).

Tape upper end of manometer tube taut to intravenous stand.

When cotton is used in manometer arm as an air filter, a needle inserted into the tubing at this point ensures a patent vent should the cotton filter become wet (see Figure 19).

Adjust stopcock to allow solution to flow into manometer arm, filling it halfway.

Adjust three-way clamp to fill remaining intravenous tubing.

4. Select vein.

Basilic. The basilic vein provides the most readily accessible route (see Figure 25). The catheter is introduced into the basilic vein and through the axillary vein, which is a continuation of the basilic. The axillary vein ends in the subclavian vein and the catheter is threaded into the right innominate to the junction of the superior vena cava.

Cephalic. Difficulties are frequently encountered when introducing the catheter through the cephalic vein. The cephalic vein enters the axillary vein at its termination; this junction may offer resistance when the catheter is

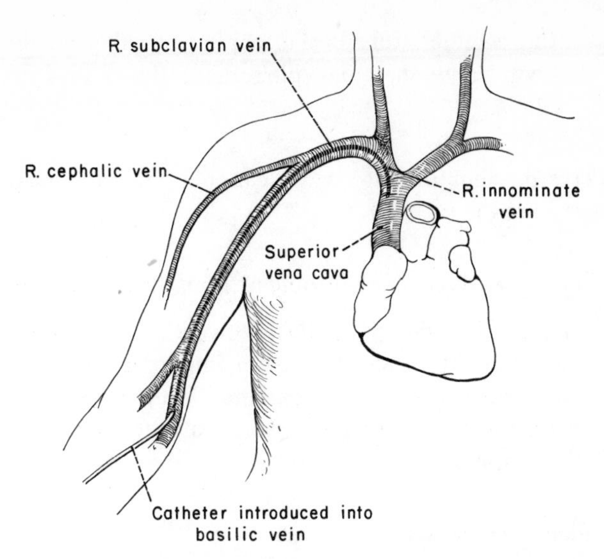

FIG. 25. Course the central venous catheter takes when introduced into the basilic vein. Notice the smooth, uninterrupted route of the catheter as it passes from the basilic vein, through the axillary vein, and into the subclavian.

inserted. Positioning the patient's arm at right angle to the body may facilitate introduction of the catheter.

5. Approximate catheter length to be introduced.

   With the catheter, measure the distance from the suprasternal notch to the anticipated puncture point.

6. Prepare site with an accepted antiseptic.

7. Inject 1% procaine subdermally to raise a small wheal.

8. Puncture the skin and fascia using a needle with a 15-gauge bore.

   Avoid puncturing the vein.

   The prepuncture prevents the sharp cutting edge of

the cannula from boring a plug of skin or subcutaneous tissue that may plug the catheter or form embolus.

9. Perform venipuncture with cannula which comes connected to the catheter.

10. Thread catheter short distance through the cannula.

    Grasp the catheter lightly with one hand while threading with the other: this is an important precautionary measure to prevent the catheter from being accidently withdrawn and possibly severed by the cutting edge of the cannula.

11. Release tourniquet.

12. Thread catheter to the premeasured distance.

13. If the venipuncture is unsuccessful, remove the needle and catheter together.

    Never manipulate catheter by withdrawing it through the cannula.

The catheter is presumed to be in the thoracic cavity when (1) manometer fluid fluctuates 3 to 5 cm during breathing, and (2) coughing and straining cause the column of water to rise [2]. It may be necessary to advance the catheter slightly farther than suggested by superficial measurement. If the catheter is inserted too far and reaches the heart, higher pressure waves synchronous with the pulse will be seen [6].

14. Withdraw cannula.

15. Slide cannula into its adapter.

16. Slide bevel protector from base of cannula to cover cutting edge.

17. Connect intravenous assembly and start the infusion.

18. Apply antibiotic ointment to puncture site.

19. Apply pressure dressing.

20. Secure the catheter.

    Place a one half inch strip of tape—adhesive up—under catheter. Cross one end tightly and diagonally over catheter. Repeat with the other end, crossing the first.

    A tongue depressor placed under needle and catheter and taped over shield, independent of the arm, protects the catheter. Tape to arm.

    Tape intravenous tubing securely to arm.

    Secure arm to armboard.

    Motion of catheter upon flexion of the arm increases the potential risk of phlebitis; a kinked catheter results in unreliable readings and leads to clogging of the lumen.

21. Inscribe on tape the date of catheter insertion.

    This will help ensure removal of catheter within a safe period of time—usually 48 to 72 hours.

Central venous pressure measurement

The pressure is usually read at half-hour or hourly intervals. The patient must be quiet, not coughing or straining, and in a supine position with the zero reading at the mid-axillary level. The procedure is as follows:

1. Turn stopcock so the central venous pressure solution flows from bottle to manometer arm.

2. When manometer level reaches 30 cm turn stopcock to stop flow from the solution bottle and direct manometer flow to the patient.
3. The fluid level will drop rapidly, reaching the reading level in about 15 seconds. The central venous pressure is measured at the high point of the fluctuation.
4. Readjust the stopcock so the infusion resumes.
5. Record measurements on Vital Signs Record.

When 5 percent dextrose in water is used for monitoring venous pressure, it may be necessary to open and flush 5 ml of the solution through the catheter at 3-hour intervals to maintain patency; dextrose may cause a rouleau to form at catheter tip as it mixes with blood, contributing to catheter plugging.

Complications

Awareness of the serious complications associated with caval catheterization and the exercising of particular caution contribute to greater safety for the patient.

CATHETER EMBOLISM. One of the serious complications is catheter embolism. In 1968 Wellman and associates [7] published a review of 37 cases of catheter embolism, in 13 of which death followed the embolism. He tabulated the causes of catheter embolism as shown in Table 10.

TABLE 10. Causes of Catheter Embolism in 37 Patients

Number of Patients	Cause of Embolism
15	Catheter severed by cutting edge of needle
6	Catheter broke, independent of the needle
4	Catheter separated from the adapter
2	Catheter severed during dressings
10	Unknown

SOURCE: Wellman et al. [7].

Special precautions should be observed to prevent catheter embolism:

1. Anchor catheter securely; if accidently severed or separated from the adapter the catheter is then anchored rather than liberated.
2. Cover the needle point with the bevel shield to prevent severing the catheter.
3. Since the shield may be dislodged, tape in place on a tongue depressor.
4. Never withdraw the catheter through the needle.
5. Know the exact length of the catheter; after removal, measure to detect immediately any lost fragments.

OTHER COMPLICATIONS. Other complications of central venous pressure measurement include the following:

1. Local thrombosis
2. Thrombosis with embolism
3. Septic thrombophlebitis with septicemia and acute bacterial endocarditis

The polyethylene catheter, because it remains flexible and elastic without the use of plasticizers, is comparatively tissue inert. After a period of time, however, local thrombosis may occur. Clot formation in the vein may be due to mechanical trauma from insertion of the catheter, from motion of the catheter within the vein, or from the chemical irritation of hypertonic solutions. Thrombosis of the vena cava and the larger veins has been known to result from sclerosing agents.

Precautions to observe are these:

1. Immobilize the arm whenever a catheter is inserted over an area of joint flexion.
2. Limit duration of time to 72 hours.
3. Maintain sterility in technique.
4. Maintain asepsis by topical application of antibiotic ointment.
5. Avoid catheterization of inferior vena cava via femoral veins.

REFERENCES

1. Bansmer, G., Keith, D., and Tesluk, H. Complications following use of indwelling catheter of IVC. *Journal of the American Medical Association* 167:1606, 1958.
2. Hallin, R. W. Continuous venous pressure monitoring as a guide to fluid administration in hypotensive patient. *American Journal of Surgery* 106:164, 1963.
3. Landis, E. M., and Hortenstine, J. C. Functional significance of venous blood pressure. *Physiological Reviews* 30:1, 1950.
4. Metheny, N. M., and Snively, W. D., Jr. Venous Pressure Measurement During Infusions. *Nurses' Handbook of Fluid Balance*. Philadelphia: Lippincott, 1967. Pp. 145, 210.
5. Russell, M. V., and Maier, W. P. The ABCs of C.V.P. measurement. *RN* 32:34, 1969.
6. Ryan, G. M., and Howland, W. S. An evaluation of central venous pressure monitoring. *Anesthesia and Analgesia: Current Researchers* 45:754–759, 1966.
7. Wellman, K. F., Reinhard, A., and Salazar, E. P. Polyethylene catheter embolism. *Circulation* 37:380, 1968.
8. Wilson, J. N., and Owens, J. C. Continuous monitoring of venous pressure in optimal blood volume maintenance. *Archives of Surgery* (Chicago) 85:563, 1962.

12.
Transfusion Therapy

WITH THE INCREASING USE OF BLOOD and its components, transfusion therapy has become an integral part of the daily treatment of patients. Administration of blood should be performed by competent, experienced, well-qualified personnel. This specialized group should be familiar with the disadvantages as well as the advantages that accompany a transfusion.

Vast improvement in methods of blood collection and storage, together with growing knowledge in the field of immunohematology, has increased the safety level of transfusion therapy; however, there is still an inherent risk with every unit of transfused blood. Both the therapist and the attending nurse should be aware of this fact and be alert to symptoms of untoward reaction.

Proper handling of the blood is vital. Contamination must be avoided; hemolysis must be prevented. The therapist must be familiar with the large variety of available blood products—their advantages, disadvantages, and the proper procedures for their safe administration.

Knowledge of the fundamental principles of immunohematology provides the nurse with a better understanding of the problems associated with blood administration. Recognition of the factors that govern red cell destruction contributes to safe transfusion therapy. This information instills in the therapist an awareness of the possibility that patients may become sensitized to the many blood factors, and of the danger which this incurs. These facts bring out clearly the necessity for screening patients for antibodies which they may develop from infused blood. Through an understanding of why bloods react unfavorably with other bloods, the therapist is keenly alert to the early symptoms of transfusion reactions.

BASIC IMMUNOHEMATOLOGY

Immunohematology is the science that deals with antigens of the blood and their antibodies. *Antibodies* (or agglutinins) are proteins in the plasma which react with specific *antigens*. They may occur naturally or may be the result of immunization against an antigen (an agglutinogen). The most important antigens in the blood transfusion are situated on the surface of the red cells.

In vitro (in a test tube) antibodies first react with their antigens by being absorbed onto the red cells (coating). The reaction may stop there or may proceed to either agglutination, in which the red cells are stuck together in clumps, or hemolysis, in which the cells burst, releasing their hemoglobin [4]. Which of these processes occurs depends upon the particular antibody involved. Coating or agglutination in the test tube is associated in vivo (in the body) with sequestration of the affected cells in the liver or spleen prior to destruction (extravascular destruction). Hemolysis in the test tube is associated with in vivo destruction of red cells in the circulation (intravascular hemolysis).

An antibody bears the same designation as the antigen with which it reacts. For instance, anti-A reacts with antigen A. A red cell antigen and its corresponding antibody are not produced in the same individual; i.e., anti-A antibody is not produced by an individual whose red cells bear the A antigen.

Blood group systems

The best-known blood group system is the ABO system, discovered by Karl Landsteiner in 1901. He demonstrated a classification of human blood based on antigens on the red cells and antibodies in the serum [4] (see Table 11.)

TABLE 11. ABO Classification of Human Blood

	Cell Antigens		Plasma Antibodies		% U.S.
Group	A	B	A	B	Populace
O	−	−	+	+	45
A	+	−	−	+	40
B	−	+	+	−	10
AB	+	+	−	−	5

In 1940 Landsteiner and Wiener discovered the Rhesus system, so called because of its relationship to the substance in the red cells of the Rhesus monkey. The antigens belonging to the Rh system are C, D, E, c, and e. Because of the ease with which antibody D is built up, typing is done to ensure that D negative recipients receive D negative blood. If a person is found to be D negative, a complete Rh typing should be done to check for the presence of C and E antigens. A person whose blood contains a D antigen is classified as Rh positive; lacking the D, C, and E antigens, Rh negative.

Eight other blood group systems have been defined on the basis of reaction of cells with antibodies: Kell, Duffy, Kidd, Lewis, MNS, P, Lutheran, and Diego. Others are under investigation. Corresponding antibodies to the blood group antigens in most of these systems are found so infrequently that they do not cause an everyday problem. When present, these antibodies may produce hemolytic reactions; once discovered, precautions must be taken to ensure that the patient receives compatible blood. When difficulty arises in cross-matching, or when a transfusion reaction occurs, these systems take on a special significance. The American Association of Blood Banks (A.A.B.B.) requires that a patient once transfused must be screened for irregular antibodies in the 48 hours preceding any further transfusions.

The term *hemolytic transfusion reaction* denotes the clinical symptoms caused when the red cells of either the recipient or the donor are destroyed in the recipient during a transfusion. Of prime importance in transfusion therapy is the assurance of ABO compatibility between donor and recipient. Since serious transfusion reactions have been reported due to transfused anti-A or anti-B antibodies, type O blood should not be used for A, B, or AB recipients. According to American Association of Blood Bank Standards [2], when a delay in blood transfusion may jeopardize life, uncrossmatched type O blood may be given to recipients whose ABO type is not known, providing certain requirements are met:

1. Levels of anti-A and anti-B are reduced by removal of at least 70 percent of the plasma from whole blood. This is the preferred method.
2. Type O whole blood is free of hemolytic anti-A and anti-B when administered to other than type O recipients.

The same requirements apply when type A or type B blood is used for type AB recipient: 70 percent plasma removed from whole blood or whole blood free of hemolytic antibodies.

OBJECTIVES OF TRANSFUSION THERAPY

There are three main objectives of transfusion therapy:

1. Maintain blood volume
2. Maintain oxygen-carrying capacity of the blood by supplying red cells

3. Maintain coagulation properties by supplying the clotting factors found in platelets and plasma

Transfusion therapy is also vital when blood exchange is imperative, as in the treatment of newborn infants with hemolytic anemia. In cardiac surgery blood is needed to prime the oxygenating pump and maintain circulation.

WHOLE BLOOD

Acid-citrate-dextrose (ACD) solution is commonly used for blood preservation and storage. Sodium citrate, by combining with ionized calcium, inhibits clotting and serves as an anticoagulant. Dextrose prolongs the life of the red cells. Acid prevents caramel formation of dextrose after autoclaving. Under controlled refrigeration of 1° to 6° C, ACD blood can be safely stored up to 21 days. This time duration is based on the standard that 70 percent of the red cells of such blood (21 days old) must be present in the blood stream of the recipient for more than 24 hours after transfusion [5].

Whole blood transfusions are indicated when an acute blood loss has occurred. The volume expanders, plasma, dextran, and albumin are useful only as a temporary measure. They lack the oxygen-carrying red cells necessary in treating hypoxia, associated with hypovolemic shock. Frequently acute blood loss requires massive transfusion.

Definite changes take place in stored blood which make age a problem for consideration when a large quantity of blood (over 6 pints) is infused in a short period of time. With the continuous metabolic changes of red cells occurring during blood storage, the potassium content of the plasma increases; potassium leaks out of the cells into the plasma. This potassium, plus that released from the intact cells, causes the plasma potassium level to rise from 7 mEq per liter the first day to 23 mEq per liter by the twenty-first day [5]. This is an important factor in the event of massive transfusions and in blood exchange of the newborn infant.

In major surgery when rapid transfusing with large quantities of blood is indicated, whole blood—as fresh as possible—is used. When the plasma potassium level reaches 10 to 15 mEq per liter, cardiac arrest and death occur [8].

Coagulation factors of the plasma and platelets are also affected by the age of the blood. In hemorrhage, when viable platelets are a consideration, fresh blood must be used. Fresh blood is also used in blood exchange in the newborn infant.

The anticoagulant can present problems. Rapid administration of citrated blood can cause calcium deficit. A damaged liver may be unable to keep up with rapid administration of sodium citrated blood, unable to metabolize the citrate ions; the citrate ions combine with ionized calcium in the bloodstream, causing a calcium deficit [8].

In conjunction with cardiac surgery, massive amounts of whole blood are required to prime the oxygenating pumps, maintain circulation, and replace blood loss. ACD blood, preferably less than 5 days old, is used for the priming of the pump. Freshly collected blood may be needed if the patient is bleeding after operation.

Packed red cells

Packed red cells are prepared by the removal of approximately 200 to 225 ml of plasma from whole blood—either by centrifuge or by sedimentation. Packed cells with a hematocrit of about 70 percent are readily transfusable; the National Institutes of Health standard is for hematocrit reading of from 60 to 70 percent. With the removal of greater amounts of plasma, difficulty is encountered upon infusion due to the resultant densely packed cells.

There are definite advantages in the use of packed red cells: reduced volume, reduced chemical content, and reduced agglutinins.

REDUCED VOLUME. Because of its reduced volume, a unit of packed cells can supply red cells without overloading the circulation—a definite advantage in patients with normal or increased blood volume and those with heart disease. Packed red cells are used for patients not in need of plasma. One unit of packed cells, in a much reduced volume, provides the same amount of oxygen-carrying red cells as one unit of whole blood.

REDUCED CHEMICAL CONTENT. The excess plasma potassium content in stored blood is reduced by the removal of plasma. Red cells can be provided for patients with kidney and heart disease without adding to the patient's hyperkalemia.

Packed cells have an advantage for patients on sodium restriction, since the sodium excess in the plasma (increased by the anticoagulant sodium citrate) is thus avoided. Packed cells also reduce hazards associated with sodium citrate, such as citrate intoxication caused by the inability of the liver to metabolize citrate.

REDUCED AGGLUTININS. Packed cells provide relatively safe low titer type O blood. Most of the plasma is removed, thereby reducing the amount of anti-A and anti-B agglutinins.

FROZEN BLOOD

The storage time for donated blood has been increased to three years or better by the process of freezing blood. This processing is accomplished through a machine, the Cytoglomerator,* invented by Charles E. Huggins, M.D. Early attempts at freezing blood proved unsuccessful because of the ice crystals which damaged the red cells. Several techniques have been developed in the past ten to sixteen years, but Dr. Huggins's method has proved the simplest and quickest.

Plasma is extracted from the whole blood. The red cells are then coated with glycerol to prevent damage from freezing and packed in disposable plastic bags. They are then frozen at −85° C, labeled, and stored until used.

Just prior to use, the plastic bag with the frozen cells is thawed in a water bath of about 40° C. The thawing time is about 3 minutes. The bag is then inserted into the Cytoglomerator for a glycerol washout of about 20 minutes. Sugar solu-

* International Equipment Co., Needham Heights, Mass.

tions are used to cause a rapid sediment of the red cells. The machine takes its name from *cyto* (cell) and *glomerator* (cluster). Three dilutions are necessary. Five pints of blood can be processed every 20 minutes by one machine.

Frozen blood offers advantages other than the long storage period. (1) It is believed that the possibility of transmitting hepatitis by transfusion of frozen blood is negligible. (2) Due to the selection of donors, frozen blood may be given to patients sensitized from previous transfusions. Type O frozen blood can safely be used as a universal donor because anti-A and anti-B antibodies are removed during washings. (3) Some surgeons believe that frozen blood plays a big part in improving results in kidney transplants; fewer of the white blood cell antigens remain to trigger the body's rejection to foreign tissue [7].

The hematocrit of frozen blood is 80—a little more than packed cells, but because of the lack of any plasma, the viscosity is less, making it easily transfusable. It may be administered rapidly to most patients.

Plasma

Plasma is the liquid content remaining after the red cells have been removed from whole blood by centrifuge. Commercially it is available in the liquid and dried state. The storage of plasma presents less of a problem than that of blood. When stored according to A.A.B.B. Standards [2], the shelf life of single donor liquid plasma in glass container is no more than 3 years, freeze dried plasma no more than 7 years, frozen plasma no more than 5 years, and fresh frozen plasma no more than 1 year.

Liquid stored plasma is prepared from ACD blood. Special precaution must be taken to avoid contamination in the preparation of plasma. A closed system under sterile conditions is used to separate plasma from red cells. Further precautions include culture of the plasma plus visual inspection.

Plasma is prepared as single donor plasma, and labeled with the specific blood group. Because plasma is a vehicle for transmitting hepatitis, the single donor plasma carries fewer risks.

Many donors are involved in the preparation of pooled plasma, thereby increasing the likelihood of viral contaminated plasma. The use of pooled plasma is to be discouraged.

Every precaution is used to reduce the risk of hepatitis. Donors are questioned for any possible history of hepatitis; this in itself is helpful, but there is no sure way to eliminate donors who may transmit hepatitis. It was thought that plasma stored for 6 months at 30° to 34° C would inactivate the virus, but cases of hepatitis have continued to appear after the use of commercially pooled plasma so stored, raising the doubt as to the effectiveness of this procedure. The use of single donor plasma, which carries less risk, is preferable, or the use of a substitute such as 5 percent albumin.

Plasma plays an important role in the treatment of burns. It supplies plasma protein and prevents shock without overloading the circulation with red cells. It may be used in emergency to correct hypovolemia. Most of the clotting factors are lost during storage, making it of little use in patients with coagulation problems.

Under ordinary circumstances when single unit plasma is used it should be compatible with the recipient's red cells. AB plasma, because it lacks anti-A and anti-B agglutinins, may be used for all ABO groups. The group O patient may receive plasma of any group. For the group A patient, only plasma taken from blood group A or AB may be used. For the group B patient, only plasma taken from blood group B or AB may be used. For the group AB patient, plasma from group AB blood only is used. In an emergency when the patient's blood group has not been determined, AB plasma is used.

Freeze dried plasma is dried plasma that has been stored in a liquid state at 32° C for 6 months before being dried [5]. It may be made from pooled plasma and used for patients of any blood type. It must be reconstituted with sterile water before use. The sterile water is packaged in a kit with the plasma. A sterile pyrogen-free filter must always be used in the administration of all plasma. Once reconstituted, freeze dried plasma should be used immediately.

Fresh-frozen plasma is beneficial to patients with inherited or acquired disorders of coagulation. Special donors with blood high in certain clotting factors are desirable. The plasma is separated from the cells and frozen within 4 hours of collection. Freezing preserves the various clotting factors, in particular factors V and VIII, to control hemorrhage in the presurgical hemophiliac.

Fresh-frozen plasma must be stored at −20° to −30° C and kept frozen until transfusion time. It is thawed in a water bath of 37° C. The fresh-frozen plasma must be administered immediately upon thawing; any delay causing a rise in the temperature of the plasma results in loss of factor VIII (antihemophiliac factor, AHF).

PLASMA COMPONENTS. *Cryoprecipitate* is a concentrate containing factor VIII (AHF) extracted from cold-thawed plasma. It was discovered by Judith G. Pool, Ph.D., Stanford University Medical Center, who began work on it in 1959. Since 1965 it has been used for treatment of hemophilia, this being the only coagulation deficiency for which it is therapeutically valuable [9].

The potency of AHF in cryoprecipitate far exceeds that in fresh-frozen plasma. Dr. Pool [9] states that approximately 6 units or 1600 ml of plasma would be necessary to raise the patient's AHF level from less than 1 percent of normal to 50 percent of normal, whereas only 55 ml or less of the concentrate produces the same results. It would take 2 hours or more to infuse the plasma but only 5 minutes to infuse the precipitate. This small volume avoids the risk of overloading circulation in patients who are not able to tolerate an increase in blood volume.

The blood from which the precipitate is taken can be reconstituted and used as whole blood or separated into components for patients other than the hemophiliac.

In the preparation of AHF, the plasma goes through a quick-freeze process. When frozen solid it is thawed at 4° C, which takes about 24 hours. The precipitate is then removed from the cold-thawed plasma.

Studies indicate that AHF levels in cryoprecipitate remain after 3 months of storage in frozen packs.

Fibrinogen, a concentrate of the fibrinogen factor, is useful in the treatment of hemorrhage resulting from a deficiency of this protein. This deficiency is most frequently seen in the obstetrical patient and at times in patients with fibrinolysin undergoing major surgery. Approximately 12 units of blood are needed to supply the amount of fibrinogen in a 2 gm unit [3]. It is stored at a temperature of 2° to 10° C in the lyophilized state.

Because the hepatitis virus is associated with fibrinogen of the plasma (hepatitis virus and fibrinogen go together during fractionation), there is increased risk to the patient infused with this product.

Fibrinogen is reconstituted with sterile distilled water—the sterile water is supplied in a kit with the fibrinogen. Care in preparation is important. Rapid shaking traps the fibrinogen particles, increasing the difficulty in reconstitution; hot water must not be used, and the fibrinogen itself must not be warmed. Administration requires a filter, preferably the set with the filter supplied with the product. Dosage varies from 2 to 8 gm, the amount depending upon individual need. Fibrinogen must be administered within 1 hour of reconstitution.

The disadvantages in the use of fibrinogen are the increased risk of hepatitis [3] and the large volume of blood needed to prepare this product.

Human albumin is prepared in a 25 percent solution containing the protein of albumin in concentrated form. Because of its low salt content, it is indicated in cases of hypoalbuminemia caused by liver and kidney disease. Albumin serves the same function as plasma. It is useful in the treatment of shock and burns without the added risk of transmitting serum hepatitis; processing by heating at 60° C for 10 hours destroys the hepatitis virus [3]. One hundred milliliters containing 25 gm of albumin require 3000 ml of blood for processing [5]. Albumin increases the osmolality of the plasma and draws fluid into the circulation, relieving hypovolemia. One hundred milliliters is osmotically equivalent to 500 ml of citrated plasma and produces a plasma volume increase of a probable 450 ml.

Human albumin is also available as a 5 percent solution in saline. Preparations contain 5 gm of normal serum albumin in each 100 ml, with the sodium content approximately that of isotonic sodium chloride solution. It is osmotically equivalent to an approximately equal volume of citrated plasma and may be used as a substitute for plasma; special processing destroys the hepatitis virus. Maximum osmotic effect is obtained with no additional fluid, while the 25 percent albumin depends for its maximum osmotic effect on additional fluids either drawn from the tissues or administered separately.

Concentrated albumin (25 percent) is sometimes diluted in parenteral solutions of dextrose, saline, or sodium lactate to obtain a less concentrated solution for patients with edema, unable to tolerate large, concentrated doses. Once mixed it must be used immediately and not stored in a refrigerator for further use. To do so could cause serious reactions from bacterial contamination. Albumin contains no preservative; once the vial is entered with a needle, it must be used immediately or discarded. The set supplied with the albumin contains a small, concealed mesh filter. *Plasma protein fraction (human)* is plasma from which the fibrinogen and much of the globulin have been removed. The preparation Plasmanate* contains 88 percent normal human albumin, 12 percent globulin, and a minimum concentration of electrolytes. It provides a substitute for plasma with the minimum risk of viral hepatitis; processing by heating to 60° C for 10 hours inactivates the virus [5]. It is indicated as a plasma expander in treatment of shock and burns.

Administration is by intravenous route, using the set provided in the package. Rate of administration and dosage is gauged to the individual and his needs. The minimum dose is usually 250 to 500 ml; rates of 1 liter per hour have been well tolerated. Untoward reactions are rare. Plasmanate should not be mixed

* Cutter Laboratories, Berkeley, Cal.

with protein hydrolysate solution or solutions containing ethyl alcohol or administered through the same administration sets.

Plasma substitute

Dextran is a plasma volume expander used for the treatment of hypovolemic shock. When introduced into the blood stream, dextran increases the osmotic pressure, draws interstitial fluid into the vessels, and increases the blood volume. It is a synthetic product with two advantages: (1) no storage problem and (2) no danger of hepatitis [8].

It is available as dextran 6 percent in normal saline solution or dextran 5 percent in water for patients requiring low sodium intake. The usual dose is 500 ml. Military hospitals and Massachusetts General Hospital use no more than 1 liter per 24 hours.

Allergic reactions to dextran are rare, but precautions should be taken. The first few milliliters of dextran should be administered slowly and the patient observed for possible reactions. These may include mild urticaria, tightness of chest, and hypotension [8]. If any such symptoms occur, the dextran must be discontinued.

The rate of flow should be ordered by the physician. Caution must be observed when dextran is administered to patients with heart or kidney disease; rapid rate may cause congestive heart failure and pulmonary edema.

BLOOD ADMINISTRATION

With the rapid advancement in transfusion therapy, responsibility for administering this vital fluid increases. Only those well versed in every phase of therapy should hold this responsibility. The patient's safety depends upon adherence to specific rules regarding safe administration. The therapist is responsible for the following:

1. Patient-blood identification. The avoidance of mistaken identity is imperative.

2. Inspection of blood prior to administration to avoid infusing the patient with hemolyzed, clotted, or contaminated blood.
3. Proper technique is necessary.
4. Close observation of the patient. Early detection of symptoms of a reaction is important.

Patient-blood identification

Patient-blood identification is of paramount importance in preventing reactions from incompatible blood. The risk of identification errors occurring from copying information onto requisitions has been reduced by the use of the addressograph. The use of triplicate requisitions also reduces the danger of identification errors. This requisition, identifying the patient, indicating amount and kind of blood and time needed, is sent to the blood bank with the blood sample. One copy is retained at Dispatch or on the ward for demand of the processed blood. The upper portion is returned with the cross-matched blood to the floor.

All personnel handling blood are responsible for checking patient-bottle identification: name and unit number of the patient, blood groups of donor and recipient with blood groups on blood container, blood numbers and expiration date. The nurse on the ward is responsible for the first check when accepting the blood.

The intravenous nurse is responsible for a repeated check. In addition the requisition is checked with the patient's chart and then with the patient himself.

The patient receiving the blood must identify himself by complete name. Identity should never be made by addressing the patient by name and awaiting his response. Errors can occur from faulty response of medicated patients.

Hospital numbers on the identification bracelet must match unit numbers on the tag to prevent errors in case of like names. Any discrepancy must be investigated and corrected before the blood is administered.

Blood must never be administered to a patient who is unable

to identify himself without some form of identification bracelet. An attending nurse may supply the identification.

Handling of blood

Blood should be administered within 30 minutes of the time it leaves the bank. The National Institutes of Health and Massachusetts state regulations require controlled refrigeration (1° to 6° C). Ward refrigeration is not controlled and contains no alarm in case of fluctuation of temperature; therefore it must *not* be used for blood storage. Present regulations require that the temperature for storing blood must not vary more than 2°. Red blood cells deteriorate rapidly when blood remains at room temperature over 2 hours. If warm blood is indicated, a special set containing a heat exchange coil should be used (see Chapter 2). Hot water must never be used to heat blood.

Blood inspections

Just prior to use, the transfusion therapist should carefully inspect the blood for abnormal color or gas bubbles which may indicate bacterial growth, and for abnormal appearance which may denote hemolysis or clotting.

Administration

Before administering the blood, the red cells should be resuspended by repeated inversion. A sterile pyrogen-free filter must be used for any blood administration. The filter should be changed often enough to prevent clogging of the filter by accumulation.

When possible, isotonic saline should be used to initiate the transfusion. Whole blood should not be hooked up in series with 5 percent dextrose in water, or run simultaneously with 5 percent dextrose in water via the Y tube; hemolysis may result. (Hemolysis does not occur when 5 percent dextrose in water solution is infused into the bloodstream, because of its rapid dilution with the blood [8].)

Hypotonic or hypertonic solutions should not be used to

dilute blood. Extreme hypotonicity causes water to invade the red cells until they swell and burst, causing hemolysis. Hypertonic solutions diluting blood result in reversal of this process with shrinkage of the red cells. Solutions containing calcium should not be used to start citrated blood; to do so could cause clotting of the blood in the infusion set.

The administration set, with a filter, may contain a chamber for compressing to expedite the flow of blood. When whole blood is needed with such rapidity that positive pressure is necessary, it should be the physician's responsibility. Great caution is necessary. Certain risks may be involved when the blood is rapidly infused: circulatory overloading with pulmonary edema, citrate toxicity, cardiac arrest, and air emboli.

Once the transfusion is initiated, the therapist should observe the patient for at least the first 5 minutes of the infusion. Many of the fatal incompatible transfusion reactions produce symptoms early in the course of the infusion. The therapist and the attending nurse share a responsibility for safe transfusion administration. They must be familiar with the various transfusion reactions, recognize adverse reactions, and know what procedure to follow.

Transfusion reactions

The following are adverse reactions which are hazards of transfusion administration.

FEBRILE REACTIONS. Chills, rapid rise of temperature, and headache are associated with leukocyte agglutinins. They appear more frequently in women who have had multiple pregnancies and in repeatedly transfused patients, i.e., patients who have had ±40 units of blood. The infrequency of the development of leukocyte antibodies may be explained by the fact that leukocytes are not well preserved in stored blood [6]. Frozen blood is an answer to the problem; white cells have been removed by the repeated washings. In addition to the symptoms indicated, when the reaction is more severe backache, nausea, vomiting, and hypotension may develop. The nurse, on observing the symptoms of febrile reaction, should stop the transfusion immediately, note vital signs, and notify the physician and the Blood Bank.

CONTAMINATED BLOOD. Reactions from contaminated blood are rare. Improved techniques in blood collection, innovation of disposable equipment, and rules governing controlled refrigeration in storage of blood have reduced the risks of contaminated blood. Careful inspection of blood prior to use may alert the therapist to contamination. Reactions are severe and may be fatal. Severe shock usually occurs at the onset. Vasopressors and antibiotics have been used to treat such reactions.

PYROGENIC REACTIONS. Chills and fever occur when substances of nonpathogenic bacterial origin are infused into a patient. They occur during or after a transfusion and recovery is usually uneventful. Disposable pyrogen-free equipment and solutions have reduced such reactions.

ALLERGIC REACTIONS. Allergic reactions are manifested by urticaria or hives and occasionally are accompanied by chills and fever. Severe reactions may occur with asthmatic symptoms, fever, and anaphylactic shock. The appearance of any of these symptoms is an indication for immediate interruption of the transfusion.

Donors with allergies or hypersensitivity to certain drugs may be responsible for some of these reactions. A donor hypersensitive to a drug may have developed antibodies against the drug; blood from the donor infused into a patient who is receiving the drug may cause allergic reactions [5].

Elimination of donors with allergies and hypersensitivity to drugs reduces the incidence of allergic reactions, but reactions still occur. Treatment consists of administration of antihistamines. Epinephrine or steroids are used in the most severe cases.

HEMOLYTIC TRANSFUSION REACTIONS. Hemolytic transfusion reactions are the most serious and may be fatal. These reactions are caused by intravascular hemolysis (rupture of red cells within the blood stream) from an infusion of incompatible blood. Blood accidently hemolyzed from improper handling may also produce hemolytic reactions when infused. Symptoms usually occur early in the course of the transfusion and include pain in the lower back and legs and tightness of the chest with breathlessness and shock. Fever may develop later and then hemoglobinuria, due to the accumulation of free hemoglobin in the blood stream.

The transfusion must be stopped at the first sign of a reaction, vital signs taken, and the physician and Blood Bank notified. A blood sample of 10 ml should be sent to the Blood Bank with the blood container. A sample of urine should be collected for detection of hemoglobin and urobilinogen, and all urine saved for observation of discoloration.

Treatment of hemolytic transfusion reactions usually consists first of combating shock by infusion of plasma and other fluids. Pressor agents may be used to treat hypotension. When kidney function is adequate, fluid and electrolytes may be necessary to maintain balance.

DANGERS FROM OVERTRANSFUSION. If the blood is infused too rapidly, a rise in the venous pressure may result. This is especially true in the aged and in patients on the verge of cardiac failure. Pulmonary edema, congestive failure, or hemorrhage into the lungs and the gastrointestinal tract may occur.

Monitoring the venous pressure guards against overtransfusion. The use of packed cells to infuse patients with normal blood volume may prevent overloading the circulation.

The patient may complain of pounding headache, constriction of chest, flushed feeling, back pain, chills, fever. The nurse should stop the transfusion and notify the physician.

CITRATE TOXICITY. Citrate toxicity may be the result of an accumulation of citrate from infused ACD blood. It occurs from rapid administration of large volumes of citrated blood or from massive transfusion to patients with liver or renal impairment. The liver, unable to keep up with the rapid administration, is not able to metabolize the citrate ions; the citrate ions combine with calcium in the blood stream, causing a calcium deficit. The normal citrate level for a healthy person is 3 mg per 100 ml. When the level exceeds 50 mg per 100 ml, symptoms of toxicity may occur. Citrate administered at the rate of 1 mg per minute increases the plasma level to 12.5 mg per 100 ml; blood pumped in at the rate of 500 ml in 5 minutes would increase citrate to this dangerous level [5].

Symptoms of excess citrate include tingling of fingers, muscular cramps, convulsions, hypotension, and cardiac arrest. Most of these symptoms are absent in the anesthetized patient, making detection of toxicity difficult.

Treatment consists of slow administration by a physician of ionized calcium such as calcium chloride.

AIR EMBOLUS. Air embolus is a hazard of intravenous and transfusion therapy. It may result from

1. Rapid emptying of blood container by application of positive pressure in a vented set
2. Blood container allowed to go dry when negative pressure exists in the vein
3. Introduction of air in process of changing bottles
4. Careless use of the Y-type administration set

The risk of air emboli has been reduced by the closed system, using the collapsible plastic container. Air pressure should not be used for rapid blood infusion; air emboli may result from tenacious bubbles in the blood becoming lodged in the pulmonary capillaries [1].

If a vented blood container is allowed to go dry and a negative venous pressure exists, air will be sucked into the recipient's circulation [5]. The arm should never be elevated above the chest level; this causes a negative venous pressure in the arm.

Care should be taken in changing bottles. If the fluid level had dropped in the administration set, the trapped air will be forced into the circulation when a fresh solution is hung. The pressure pump in an administration set should be kept filled at all times.

Air emboli can result from careless use of a Y-type administration set, or an intravenous piggybacked onto an initial intravenous setup. If the clamps on both sets are left open and the vented bottle is allowed to go dry, air is sucked into the circulation; the atmospheric pressure, being greater in the empty bottle, will cause the empty bottle to become the source of air for the air vent. Although a less obvious source of air emboli, this may cause large quantities of air to be introduced into the tubing and circulation [10].

REFERENCES

1. Adriani, J. Venipuncture. *American Journal of Nursing* 62:66, 1962.
2. American Association of Blood Banks. *Standards for Blood Banks and Transfusion Services* (5th ed.). Chicago: Twentieth Century Press, 1970. Pp. 12, 13.
3. Crouch, M. L., and Gibson, S. T. Blood therapy. *American Journal of Nursing* 62:71, 1962.
4. Fisk, R. T. *A Manual of Blood Grouping and Rh Typing Serums* (3d ed.). Los Angeles: Hyland Laboratories, 1956. Pp. 5, 8.
5. Grove-Rasmussen, M., Lesses, M. F., and Anstall, H. B. Medical progress: Transfusion therapy. *New England Journal of Medicine* 264:1034–1044, 1088–1095, 1961.
6. Hyland Laboratories. *Hyland Reference Manual of Immunohematology* (3d ed.). Los Angeles, 1965. Pp. 3–7, 36, 85–87.
7. Machine Extends Blood Storage Time. *Hospital Formulary Management*. Chicago: Clissold Publishing, 1966. P. 44.
8. Metheny, N. M., and Snively, W. D., Jr. *Nurses' Handbook of Fluid Balance*. Philadelphia: Lippincott, 1967. P. 139.

9. Pool, J. G. Precipitate from cold thawed plasma potent in therapy for hemophiliacs. *Journal of the American Medical Association* 193:27, 1965.
10. Tarail, R. Practice of fluid therapy. *Journal of the American Medical Association* 171:45–49, 1950.

13.
Hypodermoclysis

On January 26, 1966, the Massachusetts Board of Registration in Nursing passed a ruling currently in effect which states that "Hypodermoclysis administration is not a nursing function." The hospital may assume responsibility, however, and delegate the procedure to a special group of professional registered nurses whom they have certified.

Hypodermoclysis is a term used to denote an injection of fluid into the subcutaneous tissue. In recent years there has been a decrease in this method of fluid administration. Problems which once justified the hypodermoclysis have been resolved by new innovations in intravenous equipment. Controlled volume sets and precision pumps have reduced the risk of speed shock which once made slow absorption by subcutaneous tissues essential. The use of the intracatheter has reduced the frequency of infiltrations, a problem which increased the use of the clysis.

Disadvantages

Definite disadvantages and hazards are associated with the subcutaneous route.

1. Fluids are not readily absorbed when infused into the subcutaneous tissues of patients with a severely reduced blood

volume because of the accompanying peripheral collapse.

2. Many types of fluids required by patients cannot be given subcutaneously. Fluids must resemble plasma in tonicity and electrolyte composition if subcutaneous absorption is to occur. Hypertonic solutions, not absorbed, draw body fluid and electrolyte into the tissues in the infused area; this may result in a reduced fluid volume, threatening circulatory collapse. These solutions increase swelling and edema, which may cause ischemia of the skin's blood vessels with subsequent sloughing of the tissues.

3. Nonelectrolyte sugar solutions are contraindicated since they may produce circulatory difficulties such as hypotension and anuria when infused into patients with a sodium deficit, a low blood volume, or renal impairment [2]. Dextrose in water attracts body fluid and electrolyte, increasing edema in the injection area and reducing the plasma volume [3].

4. Solutions such as the gastric replacement solutions, containing a pH significantly different from the blood pH, are contraindicated for subcutaneous infusion [3]. Solutions containing alcohol are irritating and may cause sloughing of the tissues. Solutions of high molecular weight, such as albumin, are not absorbed.

Suitable solutions

The solutions considered suitable for subcutaneous administration include

0.9 percent sodium chloride injection USP
2½ percent dextrose in 0.45 percent sodium chloride USP
2½ percent dextrose in half-strength Ringer's
Ringer's Solution
Lactated Ringer's
2½ percent dextrose in half-strength lactated Ringer's

Procedure for administration

The fluid may be administered through an intravenous administration set, but to hasten the infusion the hypodermoclysis set is usually used. This is a Y-type set employing 2 needles. Each arm of the Y contains a clamp to control the rate of flow.

The area most commonly used is the outer front of the thighs between the knee and the hip [1]. A generous area of skin is thoroughly prepared with iodine and alcohol. If local anesthesia is required, 0.5 ml of procaine 1 percent may be used, provided the patient has never demonstrated a sensitivity to the drug.

The following steps should be carried out:

1. Expel all air from tubing.
2. To provide sterile dressings at injection site during infusion, pierce the center of sterile gauze sponges with each needle.
3. Prepare skin thoroughly.
4. If desired, inject procaine intradermally to raise a wheal through which the needle can be inserted.
5. Hold tissues firmly in the left hand. The needle should be inserted at about a 30 degree angle with a quick motion.
6. Check for backflow of blood to ascertain that a blood vessel has not been entered. If a blood return is obtained relocate needle in subcutaneous tissue.
7. Start fluid and regulate flow.
8. Tape needle securely.

The *rate of administration* depends upon the individual's ability to absorb the fluid and should be regulated accordingly. If necessary the flow can be completely stopped until the fluid has been absorbed. To accelerate absorption, an enzyme, hyaluronidase, is sometimes injected into the tissues or added to the infusion [3].

Cautions

The following precautions should be observed:

1. The solution should be checked carefully to prevent hypertonic solution from being administered in error.

2. The rate of flow should be checked frequently to prevent any increased pressure that may impair the circulation and cause sloughing.
3. Aseptic technique must be adhered to in order to prevent abcesses due to infection. Unlike the blood, the tissues lack the abundance of antibodies necessary to combat infection, and infection in the subcutaneous tissue spreads rapidly.
4. As edematous fluid is an excellent culture medium for bacteria, a sterile dressing should be applied following removal of the needles.

REFERENCES

1. McGaw Laboratories. *Parenteral Fluid Therapy by the Subcutaneous Route.* Technical Information Bulletin. Glendale, Cal., 1966. Pp. 1–2.
2. McGaw Laboratories. *Guide to Parenteral Fluid Therapy.* Glendale, Cal., 1963. P. 27.
3. Metheny, N. M., and Snively, W. D., Jr. *Nurses' Handbook of Fluid Balance.* Philadelphia: Lippincott, 1967. P. 116.

14.
Laboratory Tests

COLLECTION OF VENOUS BLOOD SAMPLES

Many intravenous departments are now including as one of their functions the collection of venous blood samples. Definite advantages are gained when this function is allocated to the intravenous nurse. (1) The nurse, understanding the importance of the preservation of veins for infusion therapy, is cautious in her choice of veins and in her technique in drawing blood. (2) Frequently one venipuncture permits both the withdrawal of blood and the initiation of the infusion, thereby preserving veins, reducing discomfort, and avoiding undue distress of the patient. (3) The patient-blood identification is of paramount importance in preventing the error of infusing incompatible blood. Because the department assumes responsibility in patient-blood identification in administering bloods and is aware of existing hazards, its personnel are well qualified and trained in the collection of samples for typing and cross-matching.

As the collection of blood samples by the intravenous department is a comparatively new function, the nurse is too often faced with the problem of collecting blood with little or no knowledge of the tests other than the amount of blood needed and the type of tube required. This chapter is primarily for the purpose of providing the nurse with information concerning the most commonly performed laboratory tests—their purpose, normal values, and the collection and proper handling of the specimens. No attempt is made to explain laboratory procedures.

Proper collection and handling of specimens

The collection of blood samples for certain tests must meet special requirements. Some tests call for whole blood while others require components such as plasma, serum, or cells. The proper requirement must be met to prevent erroneous or misleading laboratory analysis.

Serum "contains all the stable constituents of plasma except fibrinogen" [3] and is obtained by drawing blood in a dry tube and allowing it to coagulate. Serum is required by the majority of laboratory tests in common use.

Plasma "contains all the stable components of blood except the cells" [3] and is obtained by using an anticoagulant to prevent the blood from clotting. Several anticoagulants are available in color-coded tubes. Choice of the anticoagulant depends upon the test to be performed. Most of the anticoagulants, including sodium or potassium oxalate, citrate, and ethylene diamine tetra-acetic acid (EDTA), prevent coagulation by binding the serum calcium. Other anticoagulants, such as heparin, are valuable in specific tests but not commonly used. Heparin prevents coagulation for only limited periods of time.

Whole blood is required for many tests, including blood counts and bleeding time. Potassium oxalate is commonly used to preserve whole blood.

Fasting. As absorption of food may alter the blood, some tests depend on the patient's fasting. Blood glucose and serum lipid measurements are increased by ingestion of food. Serum inorganic phosphorous values are depressed after meals.

Intravenous solutions may contribute to misleading laboratory interpretations. Blood samples should never be drawn proximal to an infusion but preferably from the other extremity. If the solution contains a substance which may affect the analysis, an indication of its presence should be made on the requisition—for example, potassium determination during an infusion of electrolyte solution.

Hemoconcentration through venous stasis should be avoided or inaccurate results will occur in some tests. Hemoconcentration increases proportionally with the length of time the tourniquet is applied. Once the venipuncture has been made, the tourniquet should be removed. This is a simple but important precaution, ignored by many. CO_2 and pH are examples of tests affected by hemoconcentration. If the tourniquet is required to withdraw the blood, it should be noted on the requisition that the blood was drawn with stasis.

Promptness of examination. Immediate dispatch of blood samples to the laboratory is vital to the accurate determination of some blood tests; promptness in examining blood samples is necessary in the analysis of labile constituents of blood. In certain tests, such as potassium, the substance being measured diffuses out of the cells into the serum being examined and gives a false measurement. To prevent this rise in serum concentration, the cells must be separated from the serum promptly.

Special handling is required with some samples when a delay is unavoidable. Some determinations, such as the pH, must be done within 10 minutes after the blood is drawn. When a delay is inevitable, the sample is placed in ice, which partially inhibits glycolysis. Glycolysis is the production of lactic acid by the glycotic enzymes of the blood cells and results in a rapid lowering of pH on standing.

Blood gases also require special handling and must be analyzed as soon as collected. When the carbon dioxide content of serum is to be determined, the blood is placed in a tube with mineral oil to prevent the escape of CO_2. Any disturbance in the interface between the blood and the oil will permit CO_2 to escape.

Hemolysis causes serious errors in many tests in which lysis of the red cells permits the substance being measured to escape into the serum. When red cells rich in potassium rupture, the serum level rises, giving a false measurement. To avoid hemolysis, special precautions should be observed:

1. Dry syringes and dry tubes must be used.
2. Excess pressure on the plunger of the syringe should be avoided; such pressure collapses the vein and may cause air bubbles to be sucked from around the hub of the needle into the blood.
3. Clotted blood specimens should not be shaken unnecessarily.
4. Force should be avoided in transferring blood to a container or tube; force of the blood against the tube results in rupture of the cells. In transferring blood to a vacuum tube, no needle larger than 20 gauge should be used.

Infected samples. Special caution must be observed in care of blood specimens suspected of harboring microorganisms that cause infectious disease. Specimens should not be allowed to spill on the outside of containers and should be placed in a paper bag or plastic container and well labeled.

Emergency tests. Blood tests ordered as emergency must be sent directly to the laboratory. Red Scotch tape is helpful in indicating a state of emergency. Tests most likely to be designated as emergencies include amylase, blood urea nitrogen (BUN), CO_2, potassium, prothrombin, sodium, sugar, and blood typing.

Venipuncture for withdrawing blood

A venipuncture when skillfully executed subjects the patient to little discomfort. The numerous blood determinations necessary for diagnosis and treatment make good technique imperative.

The stab technique should be avoided as it too often results in through-and-through punctures contributing to hematomas. The needle should be inserted under the skin and then, after relocation of the vein, into the vessel.

The veins most commonly used are those in the antecubital

fossa. The median antecubital vein, though not always visible, is usually large and palpable. Since it is well supported by subcutaneous tissue and least apt to roll, it is often the best choice for venipuncture. Second choice is the cephalic vein. The basilic vein, though often times the most prominent, is apt to be the least desirable. This vein rolls easily, making the venipuncture difficult, and a hematoma may readily occur if the patient is allowed to flex his arm; flexing the arm squeezes the blood from the engorged vein into the tissues.

Sufficient time should be spent in locating the vein before attempting venipuncture. Whenever the veins are difficult to see or palpate, the patient should lie down. If the patient is seated the arm should be well supported on a pillow.

Complications

Hematomas are the most common complication of routine venipuncture for withdrawing blood, and they contribute more to the limitation of available veins than any other complication. They may result from through-and-through puncture to the vein or from incomplete insertion of the needle into the lumen of the vein, allowing the blood to leak into the tissues by way of the bevel of the needle. In the latter case, correction may be made by advancing the needle into the vein. At the first sign of uncontrolled bleeding, the tourniquet should be released and the needle withdrawn.

Hematomas also result from the application of the tourniquet after an unsuccessful attempt has been made to draw blood. The tourniquet should never be applied to the extremity immediately after a venipuncture.

Hematomas most frequently result from insufficient time spent in applying pressure and from the bad habit of flexing the arm to stop the bleeding. Once the venipuncture is completed, the patient should be instructed to elevate his arm; elevation causes a negative pressure in the vein, collapsing it and facilitating clotting. With cardiac patients, elevation of the arm should be avoided. Constant pressure is maintained until the bleeding has stopped. Pressure is applied with a dry sterile sponge; a wet sponge encourages bleeding. Band-Aids do not take the place of pressure and, if ordered, are not applied until the bleeding has stopped. Arms covered with ecchymoses demonstrate poor technique or haphazard manner.

Other complications of venipuncture include syncope, continued bleeding, and thrombosis of the vein. Serum hepatitis may occur if the same syringes or Vacutainers are used for multiple punctures.

Syncope is rarely encountered when the therapist is confident, skillful, and reassures the patient.

Continued bleeding is a complication which may affect the patient receiving anticoagulants or the patient with a blood dyscrasia. To prevent bleeding and to preserve the vein, pressure to the site may be required for an extended period of time. The therapist should remain with the patient until the bleeding has stopped.

Thrombosis in routine venipuncture occurs from injury to the endothelial lining of the vein while performing the venipuncture. Antecubital veins may be used indefinitely if the therapist is skillful in her technique.

Hepatitis. Special caution must be exercised in the care of needles used to draw blood from patients suspected of harboring microorganisms. Contaminated needles should be placed immediately in a separate container for disposal. A vacuum tube with stopper provides adequate protection against accidental puncture from the contaminated needle until proper disposal can be made. Any needle puncture should be reported at once.

The Vacutainer

The Vacutainer, which is replacing the syringe for withdrawing blood, has done much to increase the efficiency of the program. This device consists of a plastic holder into which screws a sterile disposable double-ended needle. A rubber-stoppered vacuum tube slips into the barrel. The barrel has a measured line denoting the distance the tube is inserted into the barrel, thus embedding the point of the needle into the stopper. The stopper is not punctured until the needle has been introduced into the vein.

After entry into the vein, the rubber-stoppered tube is pushed the remaining distance into the barrel. This forces the needle into the vacuum tube which automatically draws the blood. The tourniquet is released and several specimens may be obtained by simply removing the tube containing the sample and replacing with another tube. To avoid excess blood from dripping into the Vacutainer barrel during the process of changing tubes, the finger is pressed against the vein, stopping the flow until the new tube is inserted (see Figure 26).

If there is failure in locating the vein, removal of the tube before the needle is withdrawn will preserve the vacuum in the tube.

At times it becomes necessary to draw blood from small veins. If suction from the Vacutainer collapses the vein, difficulty will be encountered in drawing the blood. By pressing the finger against the vein beyond the point of the needle or by placing the bevel of the needle lightly against the wall of

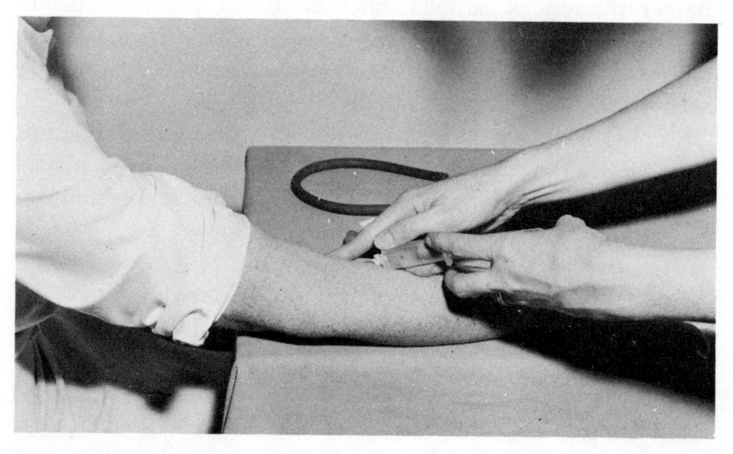

FIG. 26. When the Vacutainer is used for collecting multiple blood samples, pressure on the vein prevents blood from leaking into the barrel. (Becton, Dickinson and Co., Rutherford, N.J.)

the vein, suction is reduced and the vein allowed to fill. In the latter process, particular caution should be exercised to prevent injury to the endothelial lining of the vein. The pressure is intermittently applied and released, filling and emptying the vein. A 22-gauge Vacutainer needle is available and often used successfully when small amounts of blood are needed; the smaller needle reduces the amount of suction and may prevent collapse of the vein. A syringe is often used to draw blood from small veins as the amount of suction can be more easily controlled.

Vacutainer barrels are disposable and should be used for only one patient. There is potential danger of transmitting hepatitis when Vacutainers are reused without gas sterilization. A Vacutainer barrel free of blood gives no assurance of safety; the shaft of the needle may be contaminated by the blood sample in which it was contained. It is virtually impossible to remove the needle without touching the Vacutainer.

Drawing blood via the central venous catheter

Occasionally it becomes feasible to draw blood samples via the central venous catheter. Such occasions include difficulty in obtaining an adequate vein, cases in which the avoidance of stress is imperative, and situations in which blood tests are ordered frequently and repeatedly.

Aseptic technique is vital in preventing the introduction of bacteria into the catheter. A sterile I.V. Catheter Plug*, placed in the stopcock outlet at the time the catheter is inserted, reduces the risk of bacterial invasion.

PROCEDURE. Follow this procedure in drawing blood by way of the central venous catheter from a patient not on drug therapy:

1. Clamp off the infusion.
2. Remove catheter plug, protecting stopcock outlet, and with a sterile syringe withdraw 4 ml of blood; discard it.

* McGaw Laboratories, Inc., Glendale, Cal.

3. Using a sterile syringe, withdraw the required amount of blood. If difficulty is encountered in drawing blood samples, raise the patient's arm to shoulder level or higher. This reduces axillary pressure on the catheter.
4. Recap stopcock with a sterile plug.
5. Open clamp and flush catheter with about 5 ml of infusion fluid to maintain patency of catheter.
6. Adjust flow to prescribed flow rate.

If the patient is on drug therapy, follow the same procedure except *use a hemostat* to stop infusion temporarily; after the blood is drawn, the control clamp maintains the prescribed rate of flow without readjustment.

PRECAUTION. Patients on vasopressors may not tolerate an interruption of medication. Check with the charge nurse before stopping the infusion; extra caution may be required with a standby nurse to watch the monitor.

WITHDRAWING BLOOD AND INITIATING AN INFUSION

Drawing blood samples and initiating an infusion can be efficiently accomplished by a single venipuncture in the following way:

1. Fill intravenous set with solution.
2. Regulate the flow to a minimum rate.
3. Clamp tubing manually by kinking between third and little finger (see Figure 27).
4. Hold adapter between the forefinger and second finger, leaving the hand free for holding syringe and needle and collecting blood.
5. Draw blood.
6. Remove syringe; attach the infusion set to the needle, releasing little finger; solution will flow at the previously adjusted rate.
7. Secure needle with a piece of tape.
8. Attach syringe to needle, previously imbedded in stopper

of vacuum tube, and transfer blood. Vacuum will cause tube to fill—never apply force. Use no larger needle than 20 gauge; lysis of cells could occur.

COMMONLY USED LABORATORY TESTS

Laboratory tests are performed (1) routinely, because they point out disorders which are relatively common; (2) for diagnostic purposes; (3) for following course of a disease; (4) in regulating therapy. (See Table 12 [1] at end of chapter.)

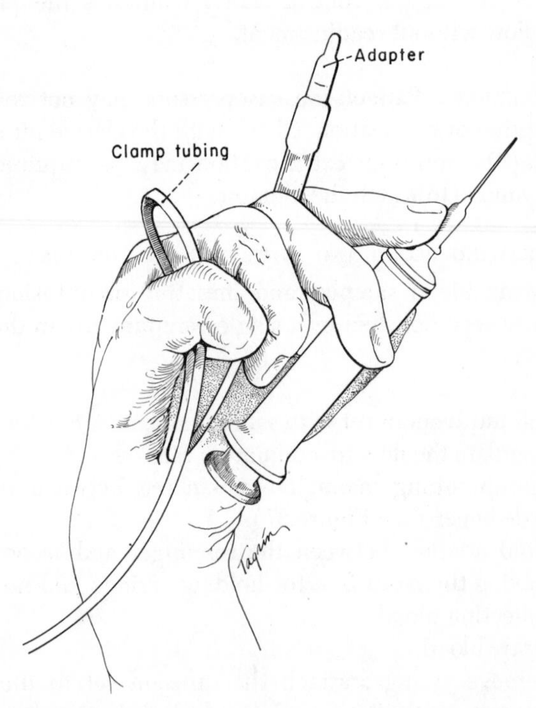

FIG. 27. Infusion tubing is clamped and held by the little finger, adapter is held between the forefinger and second finger, leaving the hand free for drawing blood sample.

BLOOD CULTURES

Blood cultures are performed to identify the microorganism present which may be producing bacteremia. Isolation of the organism is necessary to enable the physician to direct proper antimicrobial therapy. Blood cultures are performed during febrile illnesses or when the patient is having chills with spiking fever. Intermittent bacteremia accompanies such infections as pyelonephritis, brucellosis, cholangitis, and other infections. In such cases repeated blood cultures are usually ordered to be performed when the fever spikes. In other infections, such as subacute bacterial endocarditis, the bacteremia is more constant during the 4 or 5 febrile days. Usually 4 or 5 cultures are obtained over a 1 or 2 day span, and antibiotic therapy is initiated with the realization that the majority of cultures will be found to harbor the offending microorganism. If antimicrobial therapy is administered prior to the blood culture or prior to the patient's admittance to the hospital, the bacteremia may be suppressed, rendering isolation difficult [3].

Penicillinase is often ordered to be added to the blood culture medium to neutralize the existing penicillinemia and to recover the organism. Usually antibiotic therapy must be withheld to await report of culture in order to make a precise diagnosis. The penicillinase is added to the culture medium before or immediately after the blood sample is drawn.

Some bacteriology laboratories routinely culture blood under both aerobic and anaerobic conditions. If this is not done routinely and bacteremia with strict anaerobes is suspected, the laboratory should be notified, as a special culture broth is necessary.

Extreme care must be observed in preparing the area for venipuncture as the skin affords a fertile field for bacterial growth. *Staphylococcus albus,* diphtheroids, and yeast (common skin or environment contaminants) usually indicate contamination, whereas *Staphylococcus aureus* presents a greater problem by indicating either a contaminant or the presence of a serious pathogen [3].

PROCEDURE. Specimens for blood cultures are obtained as follows:

1. Prepare the skin at preposed puncture site: Cleanse a wide area with iodine. Cleanse again with 70 percent isopropanol.
2. Perform venipuncture using sterile syringe and needle.
3. Withdraw approximately 8 ml of blood.
4. Remove needle and transfer blood to culture bottle, using care not to touch neck of bottle.
5. Do not shake bottle or disturb interface on the broth of cultures drawn for anaerobic bacteria.
6. Label specimens with name, date, time, and number of culture.

Measurements of electrolyte concentration

Electrolyte imbalances are serious complications of the critically ill. Such imbalances must be recognized and corrected at once. Frequently electrolyte determinations are ordered on an emergency basis. Accurate measurement is essential and to a large degree depends upon the proper collection and handling of blood specimens.

POTASSIUM. Potassium is an electrolyte essential to body function. Approximately 98 percent of all body potassium is found in the cells; only small amounts are contained in the serum.

The kidneys do not normally conserve potassium. When large quantities of body fluid are lost without potassium replacement, a severe deficiency occurs. Chronic kidney disease and the use of diuretics may cause a potassium deficit. Adrenal steroids play a major role in controlling the concentration of potassium: hyperadrenalism causes increased potassium loss with deficiency resulting; steroid therapy promotes potassium excretion.

An elevated potassium level results from potassium retention in renal failure or in adrenal cortical deficiency. Hypoventilation and cellular damage also result in an elevated potassium level.

Because intracellular ions are not accessible for measurement, determination must be made on the serum. As the concentration of potassium in the cells is roughly 15 times greater than in the serum, the blood for potassium determination must be carefully drawn to prevent hemolysis.

Blood collection. Blood (2 ml) is drawn in a dry tube and allowed to clot or, preferably, placed under oil; oil minimizes friction and hemolysis of the red blood cells. The blood should be sent to the laboratory immediately as potassium diffuses out of the cells and gives a falsely high reading.

Normal serum range is 4 to 5 mEq per liter [2].

SODIUM. The main role of sodium is the control of the distribution of water throughout the body and the maintenance of a normal fluid balance.

The excretion of sodium is regulated to a large degree by the adrenocortical hormone, aldosterone. The regulation of water excretion is regulated by ADH (antidiuretic hormone), and as long as these two systems are in harmony, the sodium and water remain in isosmotic proportion. Any change in the normal sodium concentration indicates that the loss or gain of water and sodium are in other than isosmotic proportion [3]. Increased sodium levels may be caused by excessive infusions of sodium, insufficient water intake, or excess loss of fluid without a sodium loss, as in tracheobronchitis. Decreased sodium levels may be caused by excessive sweating accompanied by intake of large amounts of water by mouth, adrenal insufficiency, excessive infusions of nonelectrolyte fluids, or gastrointestinal suction accompanied with water by mouth.

Blood collection. Blood (2 ml) is carefully drawn to prevent hemolysis and placed in a dry tube or a tube with oil.

Normal serum range is 138 to 145 mEq per liter.

CHLORIDES. Chlorides are usually measured along with other electrolytes of the blood. The measurement of chlorides is helpful in diagnosing disorders of acid–base balance and water balance of the body. Chloride has a reciprocal power of increasing or decreasing in concentration whenever changes in concentration of other anions occur. In metabolic acidosis there is a reciprocal rise in chloride concentration when the bicarbonate concentration drops.

Elevation in blood chlorides occurs in such conditions as Cushing's syndrome, hyperventilation, and some kidney disorders. A decrease in blood chlorides may occur in diabetic acidosis, heat exhaustion, and following vomiting and diarrhea.

Blood collection. Venous blood (1 ml) is withdrawn and placed in a tube to clot.

Normal serum range is 100 to 106 mEq per liter.

CALCIUM. Calcium, an essential electrolyte of the body, is required for blood clotting, muscular contraction, and nerve transmission. Only ionized calcium is useful but, since it cannot be satisfactorily measured, the total amount of body calcium is determined; 50 percent of the total is believed to be ionized [2]. In acidosis there is a higher level of ionized calcium, in alkalosis a lower level.

Hypocalcemia (decrease in normal blood calcium) occurs whenever impairment of the gastrointestinal tract, such as sprue or celiac disease, prevents absorption. Deficiency also occurs in hypoparathyroidism and in some kidney diseases and is characterized by muscular twitching and tetanic convulsions.

Hypercalcemia (excess of calcium in the blood) occurs in hyperparathyroidism and in respiratory disturbance where carbon dioxide blood content is increased, such as in respiratory acidosis.

Blood collection. Venous blood (5 ml) is placed in a dry tube and allowed to clot. Analysis is performed on the serum.

Normal serum range is 8.5 to 10.5 mg per 100 ml [1].

PHOSPHORUS. Phosphorus metabolism is related to calcium metabolism and the serum level varies inversely with calcium.

Increased concentration of phosphorus may occur in such conditions as hypoparathyroidism, kidney disease, or excessive intake of vitamin D. Decreased concentrations may occur in hyperparathyroidism, rickets, and in some kidney diseases.

Blood collection. Since red cells are rich in phosphorus, hemolysis of the blood must be avoided. Analysis is performed on the serum; 4 ml of blood is placed in a dry tube to clot.

Normal serum range is 3.0 to 4.5 mg per 100 ml.

VENOUS BLOOD MEASUREMENTS OF ACID–BASE BALANCE

Acid–base balance is maintained by the buffer system, carbonic acid–base bicarbonate at a 1 to 20 ratio. When deviations occur in the normal ratio, a change in pH results and is accompanied by a change in bicarbonate concentration.

CARBON DIOXIDE (CO_2) CONTENT. CO_2 content is the measurement of the free carbon dioxide and the bicarbonate content of the serum, which provides a general measure of acidity or alkalinity. An increase in CO_2 content usually indicates alkalosis; a decrease indicates acidosis. This test, along with clinical findings, is helpful in surmising the severity and nature of the disorder. Measurement of pH is necessary for accuracy —a change in CO_2 does not always signify a change in pH, as pH depends on the ratio and not the CO_2 content. When the CO_2 content and pH are known, the buffer ratio can be determined.

An elevated CO_2 content is present in metabolic alkalosis, hypoventilation, loss of acid secretions such as occurs in persistent vomiting or drainage of stomach, and excessive administration of ACTH or cortisone. A low CO_2 content usually occurs in loss of alkaline secretions such as in severe diarrhea, certain kidney diseases, diabetic acidosis, and hyperventilation.

Blood collection. Blood (4 ml) is drawn without stasis; hemoconcentration may result in an erroneous report. The blood is placed in a tube under oil as contact with air permits the escape of CO_2

Normal serum range is 26 to 28 mEq per liter.

ACIDITY (pH) CONTENT. pH, a symbol for acidity, indicates the concentration of hydrogen ions in the serum. The pH becomes lower in an acid condition, such as in hypoventilation, diarrhea, and diabetic acidosis. The pH rises in an alkaline condition such as hyperventilation and excess vomiting.

Blood collection. The blood is collected *without stasis* in a heparinized 2 cc syringe; the syringe is then capped. The blood may be drawn with a scalp vein needle, the needle discarded, and the tubing tied off. The specimen is left in the syringe and packed in ice. Loss of CO_2 from contact with the air is thus avoided and excess production of lactic acid by enzymic reaction reduced.

Normal blood range is 7.35 to 7.45.

ENZYMES

AMYLASE. Amylase determination is helpful in the diagnosis of acute pancreatitis or the acute recurrence of chronic pancreatitis. Amylase is secreted by the pancreas; a rise in the serum level occurs when outflow of pancreatic juice is restricted. This test is usually performed on patients with acute abdominal pain, or on surgical patients in whom questionable injury may have occurred to the pancreas. Amylase levels usually remain elevated for only a short time—3 to 6 days.

Blood collection. Venous blood (6 ml) is allowed to clot in a dry test tube.

Normal serum range is 4 to 25 units per milliliter. The range may depend upon the normal values established by clinical laboratories, as the method may be modified.

LIPASE. Lipase determination is used for detecting damage to the pancreas and is valuable when too much time has elapsed for the amylase level to remain elevated. When secretions of the pancreas are blocked, the serum lipase level rises.

Blood collection. The test is performed on serum from 6 ml of clotted blood.

Normal serum range is under 2 units per milliliter.

PHOSPHATASE, ACID. Acid phosphatase is useful in determining metastasizing tumors of the prostate. The prostate gland and carcinoma of the gland are rich in phosphatase but do not normally release the enzyme into the serum. Once the carcinoma has spread, it starts to release acid phosphatase, increasing the serum concentration [2].

Blood collection. Blood (10 ml) is allowed to clot in a dry tube. Analysis is performed on the serum. Hemolysis should be avoided. Analysis should be done immediately or the serum frozen.

Normal serum range. (1) Male: Total, 0.13 to 0.63 Sigma unit per milliliter. (2) Female: Total, 0.01 to 0.56 Sigma unit per milliliter. (3) Prostatic: 0 to 0.7 Fishman-Lerner unit per 100 ml [1].

PHOSPHATASE, ALKALINE. Alkaline phosphatase is a useful test in diagnosing bone diseases and obstructive jaundice. In bone diseases the small amount of alkaline usually present in the serum rises in proportion to the new-bone cells. When excretion of alkaline phosphatase is impaired as in some disorders of the liver and biliary tract, the serum level rises and may give some evidence of the degree of blockage in the biliary tract [2].

Blood collection. Blood (5 ml) is drawn and the test is performed on the serum. Bromsulphalein dye should be avoided.

Normal serum range is 2.0 to 4.5 units per milliliter (Bodansky).

TRANSAMINASE

SGOT (SERUM GLUTAMIC OXALOACETIC TRANSAMINASE). SGOT is used to distinguish between myocardium infarction and acute coronary insufficiency without infarction. It is also useful as a liver function test in following the progression of liver damage or in ascertaining when the liver has recovered. Transaminases are enzymes found in large quantities in the heart, liver, muscle, kidney, and pancreas cells. Any disease which causes damage to these cells will result in an elevated serum transaminase; clinical signs and other tests are used in diagnosis.

Blood collection. The test is performed on serum from 5 ml of clotted blood.

Normal serum range is 10 to 40 units per milliliter. In myocardial infarction, the level is increased 4 to 10 times, whereas in liver involvement a high of 10 to 100 times normal may occur. The serum level remains elevated for about 5 days.

SGPT (SERUM GLUTAMIC PYRUVATE TRANSAMINASE). SGPT is another transaminase that is more specific for hepatic malfunction than SGOT.

Blood collection. The test is performed on the serum from 5 ml of blood.

Normal serum range is 7 to 25 units per milliliter [3].

SLD (SERUM LACTIC DEHYDROGENASE). The transaminase enzyme SLD is present in all tissue and in large quantities in the kidneys, heart, and skeletal muscles. Elevated serum levels usually parallel the SGOT levels. Elevation occurs in myocardial infarction and may continue through the sixth day. Elevations have been found in lymphoma, disseminated carcinoma, and some cases of leukemia.

Blood collection. The test is performed on the serum. Blood (3 ml) is collected and allowed to coagulate. Care must be taken to avoid hemolysis, as only a slight degree may give an incorrect reading. "At room temperature, hemolysis may increase the SLD activity by as much as 25 percent in 1 hour" [3].

Normal serum range is 60 to 100 units per milliliter.

Liver function tests

ALBUMIN, GLOBULIN, TOTAL PROTEIN, AND A/G RATIO. These tests may be useful in diagnosing kidney and liver disease or in judging the effectiveness of treatment. The chief role of serum albumin is to maintain osmotic pressure of the blood; globulin assists. The globulin molecule, being larger than the albumin, is less efficient in maintaining osmotic pressure and does not leak out of the blood. With the loss of albumin through the capillary wall, the body compensates by producing more globulin. The osmotic pressure is reduced and may result in some edema. A shift in the albumin–globulin (A/G) ratio assists the physician in diagnosis. The ratio is lowered in liver disease and in chronic nephritis [2].

Blood collection. Six milliliters of blood is drawn. The test is performed on the serum.

Normal serum range. (1) Total protein, 6 to 8 gm per 100 ml. (2) Albumin, 4.0 to 5.0 gm per 100 ml. (3) Globulin, 2.0 to 3.0 gm per 100 ml. (4) A/G ratio, 1.5:1 to 2.5:1.

BILIRUBIN (DIRECT AND INDIRECT). The bilirubin test differentiates between an impairment of the liver by obstruction and hemolysis. Bilirubin arises from the hemoglobin liberated from broken down red cells. It is the chief pigment of the bile, excreted by the liver. If the excretory power of the liver is impaired by obstruction, there is an excess of circulatory bilirubin and it is free of any attached protein. Measurement of free bilirubin (direct) usually indicates obstruction.

When increased red cell destruction (hemolysis) occurs, the increased bilirubin is believed to be bound to protein (indirect).

A *total bilirubin* detects increased concentration of bilirubin before jaundice is seen.

Blood collection. The test is performed on the serum from 5 ml of clotted blood.

Normal serum range is 0.1 to 1.0 mg per 100 ml [2].

CEPHALIN FLOCCULATION. This is a useful test in diagnosing liver damage, frequently detecting damage before jaundice becomes evident. It is also useful in following the course of liver disease such as cirrhosis. The serum of patients with damaged liver cells flocculates a colloidal suspension of cephalin and cholesterol, while the serum of normal patients does not clump the suspension. Abscesses and neoplasms do not damage liver cells and therefore give a negative test [2].

Blood collection. The test is performed on serum from 5 ml of clotted blood.

Normal serum range is 2+ or less in 48 hours.

CHOLESTEROL. Cholesterol, a normal constituent of the blood, is present in all body cells. Its quantity may vary from normal in various diseases. Elevation of the cholesterol level may be helpful in indicating certain liver diseases, hypothyroidism, and xanthomatosis [2].

Blood collection. The test is performed on serum from 5 ml of clotted blood.

Normal serum range is 150 to 280 mg per 100 ml.

CHOLESTEROL ESTERS. This test is helpful in estimating the amount of cellular damage in the liver and is of prognostic value in some patients with jaundice.

Blood collection. The test is performed on serum from 7 ml of clotted blood.

Normal serum range is 60 to 75 percent of cholesterol.

PROTHROMBIN TIME. The prothrombin time, considered one of the most important screening tests in coagulation studies, indirectly measures the ability of the blood to clot. It is an important guide in controlling drug therapy and is commonly used when anticoagulants are prescribed. The prothrombin content is reduced in liver diseases.

Blood collection. Venous blood (4 ml) is collected, added to the coagulant, and quickly mixed. It is important to avoid clot formation and hemolysis. The blood should be examined as soon as possible.

The *normal value* is 100 percent.

THYMOL TURBIDITY. Thymol turbidity detects damaged liver cells and differentiates between liver disease and biliary obstruction. Turbidity is usually increased when the serum of patients with liver damage is mixed with a saturated solution of thymol. Turbidity is usually normal in biliary obstruction without liver damage.

Blood collection. The test is performed on the serum from 5 ml of clotted blood.

Normal serum range is 0 to 4 units.

KIDNEY FUNCTION TESTS

CREATININE. The creatinine test measures kidney function. Creatinine, the result of a breakdown of muscle creatine phosphate, is produced daily in a constant amount in each individual. A disorder of kidney function prevents excretion and an elevated creatinine gives a reliable indication of impaired kidney function. A normal serum creatinine does not indicate unimpaired renal function, however.

Blood collection. The test is performed on the serum from 6 ml of venous blood, allowed to clot.

Normal serum range is 0.7 to 1.5 mg per 100 ml.

BLOOD UREA NITROGEN (BUN). The BUN measures kidney function. Urea, the end product of protein metabolism, is excreted by the kidneys. Impairment in kidney function results in an elevated concentration of urea nitrogen in the blood. Rapid protein catabolism may also increase the urea nitrogen above normal limits. The *nonprotein nitrogen* (*NPN*) is a similar test for measuring kidney function.

Blood collection. The test is performed on blood or serum. Blood (5 ml) is added to an oxalate tube and shaken or placed in a dry tube to clot.

Normal ranges are 8 to 25 mg per 100 ml.

BLOOD SUGARS

BLOOD SUGAR (GLUCOSE). The test for blood sugar is used to detect a disorder of glucose metabolism, which may be the result of any one of several factors, including (1) inability of pancreas islet cells to produce insulin, (2) inability of intestines to absorb glucose, (3) inability of liver to accumulate and break down glycogen, (4) presence of increased amounts of certain hormones [3].

An elevated blood sugar may indicate diabetes, chronic liver disease, or overactivity of the endocrine glands. A decrease in blood sugar may result from an overdose of insulin, tumors of the pancreas, or insufficiency of various endocrine glands.

FASTING BLOOD SUGAR (FBS). A fasting blood sugar requires that the patient fast for 8 hours.

Blood collection. Venous blood (3 to 5 ml) is collected in an oxalate tube and shaken to prevent microscopic clots.

Normal range is 70 to 100 mg per 100 ml (true blood sugar method). The normal value depends upon the method of determination. Values over 120 mg per 100 ml on several occasions may indicate diabetes mellitus.

POSTPRANDIAL BLOOD SUGAR DETERMINATIONS. The postprandial sugar test is helpful in diagnosing diabetes mellitus. Blood is drawn 2 hours after the patient has begun to eat. If the blood sugar value is above the upper limits of normal for fasting, a glucose tolerance test is performed.

GLUCOSE TOLERANCE. The glucose tolerance test is indicated

1. When patient shows glycosuria
2. When fasting or 2-hour blood sugar concentration is only slightly elevated

3. When Cushing's syndrome or acromegaly are questionable diagnoses
4. To establish cause of hypoglycemia

Blood collection. A fasting blood sugar is drawn. The patient drinks 100 gm of glucose in lemon-flavored water (some laboratories use 1.75 gm of glucose per kg of ideal body weight). Blood and urine samples are collected at 30, 60, 90, 120, and 180 minutes after ingestion of glucose.

Normal (true blood sugar) value: (1) FBS below 100 mg per 100 ml. (2) Peak below 160 mg per 100 ml in 30 or 60 minutes. (3) Two-hour value below 120 mg per 100 ml. The values are dependent on the standards used.

Blood typing

Blood typing is one of the most common tests performed on blood, being required by all donors and by all patients who may need blood. The ABO system denotes four main groups, O, A, B, and AB. The designations refer to the particular antigen present on the red cells: group A contains red cells with the A antigen, B with B antigen, AB with A and B antigens, and O red cells contain neither A nor B antigens.

When red cells containing antigens are placed with serum containing corresponding antibodies under favorable conditions, agglutination (clumping) occurs. Therefore an antigen is known as an agglutinogen, and an antibody as an agglutinin [3].

An individual's serum contains antibodies that will react to corresponding antigens not usually found on the individual's own cells. For instance, serum of group O contains antibodies A and B, which will react with the corresponding antigens A and B found on the red cells of group AB.

Although agglutination occurs in antigen-antibody reaction in the laboratory, hemolysis occurs in vivo; antibody attacks red cells, causing rupture with liberation of hemoglobin. Hemolysis results from infusing incompatible blood and may lead to fatal consequences [3].

RH FACTOR. The antigens belonging to the Rh system are D, C, E, c, and e; they are found in conjuction with the ABO group. The strongest of these factors is the D(Rh_o) factor, found in about 85 percent of the white population. Therefore the D(Rh_o) factor is often the only factor identified in Rh typing. When not present, further typing is done to identify any of the less common Rh factors before identifying an individual as Rh-negative.

Occasionally weak variants of the D(Rh_o) factor exist and are identified by means of an indirect Coombs test. These individuals, called D^u variants, are considered Rh-positive but should as recipients receive Rh-negative blood.

The serum of an Rh-negative individual differs from the main groups in that the anti-Rh antibodies are not usually present in significant quantities until the individual is exposed to an Rh+ factor, through either transfusion or pregnancy.

BLOOD COLLECTION. Venous blood is collected and allowed to clot. Usually one tube (10 ml) will set up 4 to 5 units of blood. Positive patient identification must be made before the blood is drawn; the name and number on the identification bracelet must correspond to that on the requisition and label. Identity should never be made by addressing the patient by name and awaiting his response. The label is placed on the blood tube at the patient's bedside. Once a patient has received a blood transfusion, a new specimen must be obtained on the day of transfusion to detect antibodies that may appear in the patient's circulation in response to blood previously transfused.

BLOOD GROUPING. Various methods are used in typing blood, but all involve the same general principle: The patient's cells are mixed in standard saline serum samples of anti-A and of anti-B. The type of serum, A or B, which agglutinates the patient's cells indicates the blood group. As a double check, the patient's serum is mixed with saline suspensions of A and of B red cells. The ABO group is determined on the basis of agglutination or absence of agglutination of A and of B cells.

COOMBS TEST. Not all antibodies cause agglutination in saline but merely coat the red cells by combining with the antigen, which is not a visible reaction. The Coombs test is performed to detect antibodies that cannot cause agglutination in saline; these are known as *incomplete antibodies*. Antihuman globulin serum is used. This serum is obtained by the immunization of various animals, usually rabbits, against human gamma globulin by the injection of human serum, plasma, or isolated globulin. This antiserum, when added to sensitized red cells (red cells coated with incomplete antibody), causes visible agglutination.

The Coombs test is performed in two ways. The *direct Coombs test* is performed when the patient's red cells have become coated in vivo. This test is a valuable procedure in

1. Diagnosis of erythroblastosis. The red cells of the baby are tested for sensitization.
2. Acquired hemolytic anemia. The patient may have produced an antibody that coats his own cells.
3. Investigation of reactions. The patient may have received incompatible blood that has sensitized his red cells.

The *indirect Coombs test* detects incomplete antibodies in the serum of patients sensitized to blood antigens. In contrast to the direct Coombs test involving red cells coated in vivo, the indirect Coombs uses the patient's normal red cells. When pooled, normal red cells containing the most important antigens are exposed in a test tube to the patient's serum and to Coombs serum, agglutination of the red cells occurs and indicates the incomplete antibody present. This test is valuable

1. In detecting incompatibilities not found by other methods
2. In detecting weak or variant antigens
3. In typing with certain antiserums, such as anti-Duffy or anti-Kidd, which require Coombs' serum to produce agglutination

TABLE 12. Blood, Plasma, or Serum Values

Determination	Normal Value	Material Analyzed	Minimal Ml. of Blood Required	Note	Method
Acetoacetate plus acetone	0.3–2.0 mg. per 100 ml.	Serum	2		Behre: *J. Lab. & Clin. Med.* **13**:770, 1928 (modified)
Aldolase	3–8 units per ml.	Serum	4	Use fresh, unhemolyzed serum	Bruno: *Biochem. Z.* **325**: 156, 1954 modified for UV analysis
Alpha amino nitrogen	3.0–5.5 mg. per 100 ml.	Plasma	5	Collect with heparin	Hamilton & Van Slyke: *J. Biol. Chem.* **150**:231, 1943
Ammonia	40–70 μg per 100 ml.	Blood	2	Collect in heparinized syringe; deliver *immediately* packed in ice.	*New Eng. J. Med.* **257**: 1161, 1957
Amylase	4–25 units per ml.	Serum	3		Huggins & Russell: *Ann. Surg.* **128**:668, 1948
Ascorbic acid	0.4–1.5 mg. per 100 ml.	Blood	7	Collect in heparin tube before any food is given	Roe & Kuether: *J. Biol. Chem.* **147**:399, 1943
Barbiturate	0 Coma level: phenobarbital, approximately 11 mg. per 100 ml.; most other drugs, 1.5 mg. per 100 ml.	Serum	5		Goldbaum: *Anal. Chem.* **24**:1604, 1952
Bilirubin (van den Bergh test)	One minute: 0.4 mg. per 100 ml. Direct: 0.4 mg. per 100 ml. Total: 0.7 mg. per 100 ml. Indirect is total minus direct	Serum	3		Malloy & Evelyn: *J. Biol. Chem.* **119**:481, 1937

Blood volume	8.5–9.0 per cent of body weight in kg.				Isotope dilution technic with I^{131} albumin
Bromide	0 Toxic level: 17 mEq. per liter	Serum	3		Adapted from Wuth: *J.A.M.A.* **82**:201, 1927
Bromsulfalein (BSP)	Less than 5 per cent retention	Serum	3	Inject intravenously 5 mg. of dye per kg. of body weight; draw blood 45 min. later.	Goebler: *Am. J. Clin. Path.* **15**:452, 1945
Calcium	8.5–10.5 mg. per 100 ml. (slightly higher in children)	Serum	3	Do serum protein also; BSP dye interferes.	Elliott: *J. Biol. Chem.* **197**:641, 1952 (modified) Kessler & Wolfman, *Clin. Chem.* **10**:686, 1964
Carbon dioxide content	26–28 mEq. per liter, 20–26 mEq. per liter in infants (as HCO_3^-)	Serum	3	Draw without stasis under oil or in heparinized syringe	Van Slyke & Neill: *J. Biol. Chem.* **61**:523, 1924 *Tech. Auto-Analyzer Meth.*
Carbon monoxide	Symptoms with over 20 per cent saturation	Blood	5	Fill tube to top; tightly stopper; use anticoagulant.	Bruchner & Desmond: *Clin. Chim. Acta* **3**:173, 1958
Carotenoids	0.13–0.67 units per ml. 0.08–0.40 μg per ml.	Serum	3	Vitamin A may be done on same specimen	Natelson: *Microtechniques of Clin. Chem.* 2d ed., p. 454, 1961
Cephalin flocculation	2+ or less in 48 hr.	Serum	1		Hanger; *J. Clin. Invest.* **18**:261, 1939
Ceruloplasmin	27–37 mg. per 100 ml.	Serum	2		Ravin: *J. Lab. Clin. Med.* **58**:161, 1961
Chloride	100–106 mEq. per liter	Serum	1		Modification of Schales & Schales: *J. Biol. Chem.* **140**:879, 1941
Cholesterol	150–280 mg. per 100 ml.	Serum	2		Babson et al.: *Clin. Chim. Acta* **7**:800, 1962

TABLE 12—*Continued*

Determination	Normal Value	Material Analyzed	Minimal Ml. of Blood Required	Note	Method
Cholesterol esters	60–75 per cent of cholesterol	Serum	2		Creech & Sewell: *Analytical Biochem.* **3**:119, 1962
Cholinesterase (pseudocholinesterase)	0.5 pH unit or more per hour	Serum	1		Michel: *J. Lab. & Clin. Med.* **34**:1564, 1949
	0.7 pH unit or more per hour for packed cells	Packed cells	1		
Congo-red test	More than 60 per cent retention in serum	Serum	5	Inject 10 ml. of 1 per cent Congo-red solution intravenously; draw blood from arm not injected 4 and 60 min. later.	Unger et al.: *J. Clin. Invest.* **27**:111, 1948
Copper	Total: 100–200 μg per 100 ml.	Serum	3		Landers et al.: *Am. J. Clin. Path.* **29**:590, 1958
Creatine phosphokinase (CPK)	0–4 units	Serum	3	Immediately separate & freeze serum	Kuby et al.: *J. Biol. Chem.* **210**:65, 1954
Creatinine	0.7–1.5 mg. per 100 ml.	Serum	3		*Tech. AutoAnalyzer Meth.*
Cryoglobulins	0	Serum	8	Collect and transport at 37° C.	Barr et al.: *Ann. Int. Med.* **32**:6, 1950 (modified)
Dilantin	Therapeutic level, 1–11 μg per ml.	Serum	5		Dill et al.: *J. Pharmacol. & Exper. Therap.* **118**: 270, 1956
Doriden (Glutethimide)		Serum	5		Rieder & Zervas, *Am. J. Clin. Path.* **44**:520

Ethanol	0.3–0.4 per cent, marked intoxication; 0.4–0.5 per cent, alcoholic stupor; 0.5 per cent or over, alcoholic coma.	Blood	2	Collect in oxalate & refrigerate	Natelson: *Microtechniques of Clin. Chem.* 2d ed. p. 208, 1961
Glucose	Fasting: 70–100 mg. per 100 ml.	Blood	2	Collect with oxalate-fluoride mixture. Micromethod: add 0.1 ml. of blood to 1.9 ml. of 0.01 per cent sodium fluoride solution	*Tech. AutoAnalyzer Meth.* Huggett & Nixon: *Lancet* **2**:368, 1957 (modified)
Iodine (protein bound)	3.5–8.0 μg per 100 ml.	Serum		Avoid iodide therapy, x-ray contrast media and iodine on skin	Leffler: *Am. J. Clin. Path.* **23**:483, 1953 (modified) Benotti and Benotti: *Clin. Chem.* **9**:408, 1963
(butanol extractable)	3–6.5 μg per 100 ml.	Serum	8	Avoid x-ray contrast media	Mann & Bondy: *J. Clin. Endocr.* **173**:317, 1957
Iron	50–150 μg per ml. (higher in males)	Serum	5	Shows diurnal variation, higher in a.m.	Landers et al.: *Am. J. Clin. Path.* **29**:590, 1958
Iron-binding capacity	Serum iron equals approximately 33 per cent of capacity	Serum	5		Scalata & Moore: *Clin. Chem.* **8**:360, 1962
Lactic acid	0.6–1.8 mEq. per liter	Blood	2	Use special bottle with iodoacetate; draw without stasis; patient must be fasting and at complete rest.	Rosenberg & Rush: *Clin. Chem.* **12**:299, 1966 (modified)
Lactic dehydrogenase	60–100 units per ml.	Serum	2	Unsuitable if hemolyzed	Wacker et al.: *New Eng. J. Med.* **255**:449, 1956

TABLE 12—*Continued*

Determination	Normal Value	Material Analyzed	Minimal Ml. of Blood Required	Note	Method
Lipase	Under 2 units per ml.	Serum	3		Comfort & Osterberg: *J. Lab. & Clin. Med.* **20**:271, 1934
Lipid partition:					
Cholesterol	150–280 mg. per 100 ml.	Serum	20	Use fasting serum	Babson et al.: *Clin. Chim. Acta* **7**:800, 1962
Cholesterol esters	60–75 per cent of cholesterol				
Phospholipids	9–16 mg. per 100 ml. as lipid phosphorus				Fiske & SubbaRow: *J. Biol. Chem.* **66**:2, 1925
Total fatty acids	190–420 mg. per 100 ml.				Stoddard & Drury: *J. Biol. Chem.* **84**:741, 1929
Neutral fat	0–200 mg. per 100 ml.			Calculated from above values	
Magnesium	1.5–2.5 mEq. per liter	Serum	2		Spare: *Am. J. Clin. Path.* **37**:232, 1962
Methanol	0	Blood	5	May be fatal as low as 115 mg. per 100 ml.; collect in oxalate.	Natelson: *Microtechniques of Clin. Chem.* 2d ed., p. 298, 1961
Osmolality	285–295 milliosmoles per kg. H_2O	Serum	5	In uremia BUN should be done to apply a correction	Crawford & Nicosia: *J. Lab. & Clin. Med.* **40**:907, 1952
Oxygen saturation (arterial)	96–100 per cent	Blood	3	Deliver in sealed heparinized syringe packed in ice	Gordy & Drabkin: *J. Biol. Chem.* **227**:285, 1957
pCO_2	35–45 mm. of mercury	Blood	5	Collect and deliver in sealed heparinized	By CO_2 electrode; also Van Slyke & Sendroy:

				in sealed heparinized syringe; deliver packed in ice.	
pO_2	75–100 mm. of mercury (dependent on age)				Oxygen electrode
Pepsinogen	200–425 units per ml.	Plasma or serum	4		Mirsky et al.: *J. Lab. & Clin. Med.* **40**:17, 1952
Phenylalanine	0–2 mg. per 100 ml.	Serum	0.4		Cullay et al.: *Clin. Chem.* **8**:266, 1962 (modified)
Phosphatase (acid)	Male — Total: 0.13–0.63 Sigma unit per ml. Female — Total: 0.01–0.56 Sigma unit per ml.	Serum	1	Must always be drawn just before analysis or stored as frozen serum; avoid hemolysis.	Bessey et al.: *J. Biol. Chem.* **164**:321, 1946
	Prostatic: 0–0.7 Fishman–Lerner unit per 100 ml.				Babson et al.: *Clin. Chim. Acta* **13**:264, 1966
Phosphatase (alkaline)	2.0–4.5 Bodansky units per ml. (infants to 14 units; adolescents to 5 units)	Serum	1	BSP dye interferes	Bessey et al.: *J. Biol. Chem.* **164**:321, 1946
Phosphorus (inorganic)	3.0–4.5 mg. per 100 ml. (infants in 1st year up to 6.0 mg. per 100 ml.)	Serum	2	Obtain blood in fasting state; serum must be separated promptly from cells.	Fiske & SubbaRow: *J. Biol. Chem.* **66**:375, 1925. Adapted for *Tech. AutoAnalyzer Meth.*
Potassium	3.5–5.0 mEq. per liter	Serum	2	Serum must be separated promptly from cells (within 1 hr.)	Flame photometry
Protein: Total	6.0–8.0 gm. per 100 ml.	Serum	1	Patient should be fasting; avoid BSP dye.	Refractometry (American Optical Co.)
Albumin	4.0–5.0 gm. per 100 ml.	Serum	1		Keyser: *Clin. Chim. Acta* **6**:445, 1961 (modified)

TABLE 12—*Continued*

Determination	Normal Value	Material Analyzed	Minimal Ml. of Blood Required	Note	Method
Globulin	2.0–3.0 gm. per 100 ml.			Globulin calculated	Gornall et al.: *J. Biol. Chem.* **177**:751, 1949 (modified)
Paper electrophoresis:	Per cent of total protein	Serum	1	Quantitation by densitometry	Kunkel & Tiselius: *J. Gen. Physiol.* **35**:89, 1951; Durrum: *J. Am. Chem. Soc.* **72**:2943, 1950
Albumin	50–60				
Globulin:					
$Alpha_1$	5–8				
$Alpha_2$	8–13				
Beta	11–17				
Gamma	15–25				
Pyruvic acid	0–0.11 mEq. per liter	Plasma	2	Use special iodoacetate tube; avoid stasis.	Rosenberg & Rush: *Clin. Chem.* **12**:299, 1966
Salicylate:	0	Plasma	5	Collect in heparin or oxalate	Keller: *Am. J. Clin. Path.* **17**:415, 1947
Therapeutic	20–25 mg. per 100 ml.; 35–40 mg. per 100 ml.; to age 10 yr.				
Toxic	Over 30 mg. per 100 ml. over 20 mg. per 100 ml. after age 60.				
Sodium	136–145 mEq. per liter	Serum	2		Flame photometry
Sulfate	0.5–1.5 mg. per 100 ml.	Serum	3	Avoid hemolysis	Letonoff & Reinhold: *J.*

Sulfonamide	0	Blood or serum	2	Value given as unconjugated unless total is requested	Bratton & Marshall: *J. Biol. Chem.* **128**:537, 1939
Thymol: Flocculation Turbidity	Up to 1 + in 24 hr. 0–4 units	Serum	1	Checked with phosphate buffer of higher molarity to rule out false-positive reaction	Maclagen: *Nature* **154**: 670, 1944
Transaminase (SGOT)	10–40 units per ml.	Serum	1		Karmen et al.: *J. Clin. Investigation* **34**:126, 1955
Urea nitrogen (BUN)	8–25 mg. per 100 ml.	Blood or serum	1	Urea = BUN × 2.14 Use oxalate as anticoagulant	Skeggs: *Am. J. Clin. Path.* **28**:311, 1957 (modified)
Uric acid	3.0–7.0 mg. per 100 ml.	Serum	2	Serum must be separated from cells at once and refrigerated	Folin: *J. Biol. Chem.* **101**: 111, 1933. Adapted for *Tech. AutoAnalyzer Meth.*
Vitamin A	0.5–2.0 units per ml. (0.15–0.6 μg per ml.)	Serum	3		Natelson: *Microtechniques of Clin. Chem.* 2d ed., p. 451, 1961
Vitamin A tolerance test	Rise to twice fasting level in 3 to 5 hr.	Serum	3	Samples taken fasting and at intervals up to 8 hr. after test dose	Josephs: *Bull. Johns Hopkins Hosp.* **65**:112, 1939

SOURCE: Prepared by: Mary Zervas, B.S., H. George Hamacher, M.S., and Olive Holmes, B.S., supervisors, and Sidney V. Rieder, Ph.D., chief of Chemistry Laboratory; M. Althea King, chief technologist, Clinical Laboratories; and William S. Beck, M.D., director of Clinical Laboratories and chief of Hematology Unit, Massachusetts General Hospital.

For values in newborn infants refer to Smith, C. A. *The Physiology of the Newborn Infant.* 3rd edition. Springfield, Ill.: Charles C Thomas, 1959.

Reprinted from the *New England Journal of Medicine* (276:167–174 [January 19], 1967) with revisions by the Chemical Laboratory of Massachusetts General Hospital.

4. In detecting antiagglutinins produced by exposure during pregnancy

BLOOD VOLUME DETERMINATION

Blood volume determinations are extremely valuable in (1) hypotension, when the origin is unknown; (2) massive fluid replacement, when circulatory overload is a hazard; and (3) anuria or oliguria, when questionable cause is dehydration.

The patient is injected with radioactive isotopes and the computation is done by the Volemetron—a precise automatic instrument that gives blood volume determinations within 15 minutes to an accuracy of 5 percent or better.

The Volemetron switch is set for adult, or for child if the blood volume is suspected to be less than 2.5 liters. The dosage, 1 ml of radioiodinated serum albumin, prepackaged in its own disposable syringe, is placed in the center well of the Volemetron. When the switch is turned the machine automatically measures and stores the value of the total dosage in its memory. If the dosage is incorrect, a yellow light indicates a weak or outdated dosage; a red light, a dosage too strong.

Venous blood is drawn for a control (8 ml for adult, 2 ml for child). The syringe is removed from the needle and replaced by the dosage syringe, utilizing one venipuncture. The isotopes are injected, the needle removed, aspirated, and discarded. The cap is replaced on the syringe. The sample of blood is transferred to a special tube marked "pre-mixed."

The empty dose syringe is returned to the instrument for a measurement of the residual. The machine automatically counts the residual isotopes, subtracts them from the dose given, and stores in memory the amount received by the patient.

After a 10-minute interval the second blood specimen is drawn from a different vein and placed in the "post-mix" tube.

The premix and postmix samples are placed in the appropriate wells. The machine automatically computes the volume, having subtracted any activity due to previous isotope administration in the premix sample. The premix sample may also be used for hematocrit determination, if desired.

REFERENCES

1. Castleman, B., and McNeely, B. Case records of the Massachusetts General Hospital: Normal laboratory values. *New England Journal of Medicine* 276:167–174, 1967.
2. Garb, S. *Laboratory Tests in Common Use* (4th ed.). New York: Springer Publishing, 1966. Pp. 28–94.
3. Page, L., and Culver, P. *A Syllabus of Laboratory Examinations in Clinical Diagnosis*. Cambridge, Mass: Harvard University Press, 1960. Pp. 22–24, 217, 260, 423, 447, 469, 550.

15. Levin Tubes

LEGAL STATUS OF THE NURSE

On December 23, 1964, the Massachusetts Board of Registration in Nursing passed a ruling currently in effect that states, "Insertion of Levin tube is a medical function that cannot be performed by a nurse." Each state may have its own rulings, and in some states the nurse practice acts relating to the definition of nursing are broad in wording and do not refer to specific procedures.

If the policy of a hospital is contrary to the ruling of the state, the hospital usually assumes responsibility and delegates the procedure to a special group of professional registered nurses whose competence has been established. The insertion of Levin tubes is becoming an added function of many intravenous departments. However, insertion of Levin tubes on patients with esophageal varices, aortic aneurysms, or severe hypertension should not be the responsibility of the nurse [2].

IMPORTANCE OF THE STOMACH TUBE

Although the passage of a Levin tube is an uncomfortable procedure for the patient, it plays a major role in the diagnosis of certain conditions and aids in the medical and surgical management of some diseases of the stomach.

Diagnostic tests

The following diagnostic tests require the use of the Levin tube:

1. *Gastric analysis* determines the degree of acidity of gastric contents.
2. *Cytology examination* aids in the diagnosis of gastric carcinoma.
3. *Acid-fast test* detects tubercle bacilli by aspirating stomach contents to recover swallowed sputum.
4. *Hollander test* demonstrates the integrity of the vagus nerve—usually after vagotomy.

Aid to treatment

Gastric aspiration is carried out by means of the Levin tube

1. To relieve dilatation of the stomach in conditions of intestinal obstruction or diabetic coma
2. To relieve distention and dilatation postoperatively
3. To empty stomach completely before surgery or gastric x-rays
4. For removal of ingested toxic substances

For patients unable to take nourishment by mouth, the Levin tube is used as a method of feeding.

USE OF THE LEVIN TUBE

The Levin tube usually has a catheter tip and is available in rubber or plastic in sizes from 12 to 18, French scale. Markings on the tube indicate 18, 22, 26, and 30 inches from the catheter tip. The tube may be introduced through the nose or the mouth, but the nasal route is preferable. Introduction through the mouth causes the tube to come in contact with the soft palate, inducing considerable gagging [2].

Equipment

Before entering the patient's room, the nurse should assemble complete equipment. The tray should be covered so as not to upset the patient. Necessary equipment consists of

1. Levin tube in good condition, clean and with the lumen patent
   a) If the tube is rubber, immerse in ice water to achieve a proper degree of coldness to make it more comfortable for the patient to swallow.
   b) Do not immerse plastic tube in ice as ice will make it stiff and nonpliable.
2. Lubricant
3. Glass of water with drinking tube
4. Aspirating syringe, preferably barrel-plunger type, large 50 cc size
5. Two emesis basins
6. Rubber sheet with a clean sheet to cover it
7. Adhesive tape
8. If a large fluid return is expected, a measured pitcher
9. If the stomach is to be lavaged, a large pitcher of warm water

Procedure

The patient should be told the necessity of the procedure. Explicit explanations should be given as to (1) what is to be done, and (2) what the patient should expect. In this procedure the patient is sitting upright in bed with head resting on a pillow. Explain that

1. The tube will be introduced through the nose to the back of the throat.
2. He will be given a glass of water with a drinking tube.
3. When the nasal tube is felt in the back of the throat, the water should be swallowed.

Carry out the procedure in the following steps:

1. Lubricate 5 to 10 cm (2 to 4 inches) of the tube with water-soluble lubricant.
2. Gently insert the catheter tip into a patent nostril.
3. Introduce the tube until it touches the posterior nasopharynx.
4. Ask patient to swallow.
   Move tube slowly so that its motion coincides with swallowing. In this way it is introduced through the esophagus without kinking back of the uvula and without causing retching and vomiting.
5. Advance tube to the second marking (about 55 cm). This usually places the tip within the stomach.
6. Tape tube to nose to hold in place and prevent discomfort of a back-and-forth motion.
7. Aspirate contents completely.
   Often a nasal tube becomes obstructed during aspiration. This may give the false indication that the stomach is empty, whereas the openings in the tube may be up against the stomach wall or small particles of food may be plugging the lumen. A small amount (20 ml) of warm water will clear the obstruction for further aspirating; aspiration of more fluid than that introduced will show that the stomach is not completely empty.
8. Note the quantity and quality of the residual (color, odor, presence of mucus, food, blood, or bile) and record in patient's chart.

Insertion of levin tube in unconscious patients

Because the unconscious patient cannot cooperate in swallowing the tube, special care is required to prevent the tube from entering the trachea and bronchials.

PROCEDURE. Carry out the procedure as follows:

1. If possible, raise the patient to a near-sitting position.
2. Insert tube into nostril and advance tube cautiously. Sometimes stroking the throat will incite the reflex of swallowing.
3. If patient starts choking, the tube could be entering the trachea. Immerse the end of the tube in water: if air bubbles arise at each expiration the tube should be removed and another attempt made.
4. Make positive proof of the tube's position in the stomach before introducing fluid or before leaving the patient:
   a) Aspirate for stomach contents.
   b) Place a stethoscope on the stomach and introduce 20 cc of air into the tube; a loud pop will be heard if the tube is within the stomach.

Gastric analysis

Gastric analysis is a diagnostic test performed to determine the degree of acidity of the stomach contents. If an ulcer is present, the degree of acidity may be greater than normal. In cases of gastric carcinoma or pernicious anemia, the degree of acidity may be decreased or acidity may be absent altogether [1].

Gastric analysis requires the stomach to be in a fasting state. The patient receives nothing by mouth after the evening meal; the procedure is usually carried out in the morning. As water dilutes the stomach contents, only a minimum amount should be swallowed with the tube. Gastric contents contaminated with saliva and duodenal contents will be affected in the degree of acidity—it is important that the tube be within the stomach [2]. Gastric juice that is bile-stained indicates that alkaline duodenal contents have flowed back into the stomach. After the tube has been introduced into the stomach, the patient should expectorate all saliva to prevent contamination of gastric secretion [2].

Use gentle suction when aspirating stomach contents. Vigorous suction may cause bleeding or cause the tube to be sucked against the gastric mucosa, obstructing the lumen of the tube.

FASTING GASTRIC CONTENTS. Aspirate entire stomach contents. Two to three drops of Töpfer's reagent may be added to the specimen to demonstate free hydrochloric acid. Red color indicates the presence of free acid. If this screening test indicates no acid, the physician may order test meals or 7 percent alcohol to produce mild stimulation [2].

If ordered, alcohol (ethanol) 7 percent, 50 ml, is instilled in the tube. A second specimen is taken about one half hour later.

If maximal stimulation of the parietal cells is necessary, the physician will usually order parenteral administration of histamine. Usually 0.01 mg of histamine base per kilogram of body weight is injected subcutaneously [2]. A specimen is taken about one half hour after the histamine injection. The tube is removed.

Histamine is contraindicated in paroxysmal hypertension and in patients who have a history of asthma. As histamine stimulates gastric secretion, it should not be given before a gastric x-ray, which requires an empty stomach.

Acid-fast test

The acid-fast test is performed on fasting patients, usually on 3 consecutive days, to detect the presence of tubercle bacilli. In handling specimens care should be taken to prevent the spread of infectious material. The entire contents of the stomach are aspirated and placed in a container—usually a glass jar with a screw top. The specimen is then placed in a paper bag, labeled to alert personnel of possible infectious material, and sent to the bacteriology laboratory.

Cytology examination

Cytology tests are performed by specially trained personnel to detect the presence of carcinoma cells. The fasting specimen, free of food contamination, is analyzed shortly after recovery to prevent digestion of cells.

REFERENCES

1. Garb, S. *Laboratory Tests in Common Use* (4th ed.). New York: Springer Publishing, 1966. Pp. 142–144.
2. Page, L., and Culver, P. *A Syllabus of Laboratory Examinations in Clinical Diagnosis*. Cambridge, Mass.: Harvard University Press, 1960. Pp. 386–389.

16.
Organization of an Intravenous Department

THE INTRAVENOUS DEPARTMENT

Because the functions performed by the Intravenous Department are not classified as nursing procedures and because the department fulfills an important part of the blood bank functions, the responsibility of this department may properly be allocated to the Director of the Blood Bank.

SELECTION OF PERSONNEL

The intravenous nurse is a registered nurse who is especially hired and trained for this specialized work. Because of its speciality and the responsibility that goes with it, the success of the department depends on the selection of its personnel. Not all nurses are successful as intravenous nurses.

The nurse must be conscientious. She will be drawing blood samples and giving transfusions where carelessness could mean a patient's life. The conscientious nurse will realize the importance of her job, the importance of being accurate, and the importance of careful patient identification. Her duties include mixing and administering drugs which, given intravenously, act rapidly. There is no margin for error.

Cooperation and teamwork are essential to the success of the department. No one individual's job is finished until the entire department has completed its work. One nurse may become involved in an emergency in which her time is utilized. There must be teamwork, a readiness and willingness to help out and accomplish the work.

Mental and emotional stability play an important part in the nurse's success as an intravenous therapist. Manual dexterity, necessary in administering an intravenous infusion, is greatly affected by the mental and emotional attitude of the nurse. The performance of few procedures is so easily affected by stress as is the execution of a difficult venipuncture.

An understanding and pleasant personality are other assets necessary to the success of the individual and the department. The nurse has unpleasant functions to perform. These unpleasant tasks are better tolerated by the patient if the nurse is understanding and congenial.

She must be tactful. The nurse works in close conjunction with the hospital nursing staff, the blood bank, the various laboratories, and the patient. Her attitude and her personality could do much to impair the harmony of these departments.

The nurse in charge of the Intravenous Department, who must assume responsibility for teaching, training, and the successful functioning of this department, should have a voice in selecting its personnel.

FUNCTIONS OF AN INTRAVENOUS DEPARTMENT

An intravenous department plays an important role in the services of a hospital. The knowledge, skill, and experience of these specially trained nurses add to the safety of the blood bank program. The administration of intravenous solutions and the collection of blood samples, performed simultaneously, do much to alleviate the anxiety of the patient and to preserve the veins. The nurses, by mixing and administering intravenous drugs and by performing other duties, relieve the doctors for their more specialized work.

The functions that are the responsibility of an intravenous

department may be many and varied. They may include the following:

1. Administration of parenteral fluids
2. Preparing and administering drugs in solution
3. Administration of blood
4. Bleeding donors
5. Bleeding patients under supervision of the physician
6. Administering hypodermoclysis
7. Collection of venous blood samples for all laboratories: chemistry, bacteriology, hematology, blood bank, and so on. This includes:
   a) Collection of blood samples routinely from all surgical admissions for typing and grouping in the blood bank
   b) Knowledge of the requirements of the various laboratory tests, including the proper collection and handling of blood samples
8. Administering Levin tubes for therapy and for diagnostic tests
9. Computing blood volumes by means of the Volemetron

TEACHING PROGRAM

The department must have a teaching program in which selected nurses are trained as intravenous therapists. This is on-the-job training. The new therapist should spend sufficient time in training with the team before assuming responsibility. Special emphasis should be placed on identification of patients and careful checking of requisitions and labels to prevent serious errors.

SETTING UP AN INTRAVENOUS DEPARTMENT

In organizing an intravenous department, the functions to be performed by this department must first be classified. If the department is to perform all functions, the work load should start at a reasonable level. By so doing the problems that may arise on initiating such a program may be met and remedied, and the success of the department may be guaranteed from the onset. It may be desirable to start by performing only a few designated functions, such as parenteral administration of fluids and bloods. After this program has been successfully organized, other functions may be added.

Before this department can go into operation, the hospital nursing staff must first be educated as to its functions.

Call system

A system for receiving calls must be organized with special emphasis on emergency calls. Some systems work to better advantage than others under various conditions. The size of the hospital, number of patients, size and location of the department, and the functions to be performed must be taken into consideration on deciding which system would be most adaptable.

REQUISITIONS. Requests for parenteral administrations and other functions may be filled out on requisitions and sent to the department. This system contains drawbacks because of the added paper work, lost time involved, and the necessity of the intravenous therapist's having to return to the department to pick up the requisitions. It may prove successful in smaller hospitals where calls are not as numerous and where the nurses are stationed in the blood bank or laboratory.

PAGE SYSTEM. The page operator lists the floor extensions as they are received. The intravenous nurse calls in every half hour and picks up her calls. Any emergency call may be put through by means of voice page or by means of a pagemaster.

ROUTINE ROUNDS. Routine rounds may be made twice a day by the intravenous therapist. The requests for services are listed on a clipboard with the patient's name and room number. When orders have been filled they are checked off by the intravenous therapist. One nurse in each building is equipped with a pagemaster. This is used only for emergency calls or requests that must be performed before the second rounds, or after rounds are completed.

This system involves less expenditure of time by the nursing staff. It eliminates the necessity for placing calls or sending out requisitions. The intravenous department is freed from unnecessary phone calls. The charge nurse, with a glance at the board, immediately knows what procedures have been performed.

PREPARATION OF EQUIPMENT

Setting up the necessary equipment for procedures to be performed must be allotted to either the nursing staff or the intravenous department.

PREPARATION OF EQUIPMENT BY INTRAVENOUS DEPARTMENT. When preparation of equipment becomes the responsibility of the intravenous department, an equipment cart must be provided on each floor. This cart carries all necessary equipment for parenteral administration:

- Intravenous solutions
- Intravenous sets
- Armboards
- Poles
- Levin tubes
- Tourniquet
- Bandage
- Adhesive tape
- Alcohol
- Syringes
- Sterile sponges

The nurse checks the orders directly from the doctor's order book. By means of the equipment cart, she sets up the procedures and initiates each order as she continues rounds.

PREPARATION OF EQUIPMENT BY THE NURSING STAFF. The nurse distributes necessary equipment, solution, set, armboard, and pole for parenteral fluids or a tray containing Levin tube equipment. The intravenous nurse carries a prep tray. This system automatically places a double check on solutions and medications ordered. It saves time. If each nurse is responsible for setting up the necessary equipment for her patient, little time is lost by her, whereas a great deal of time is utilized by the intravenous therapist in preparing all patients. This system eliminates the necessity for an equipment cart on each floor.

Cooperation of interdepartmental personnel

Before this department starts to function, a thorough explanation must be made to the staff of doctors, for only with cooperation in every department will success be guaranteed. The doctors should be requested to cooperate by writing intravenous orders early—before 9 A.M. when at all possible. This will assure the physician of his orders' being initiated at a reasonable hour. This is particularly important when the Intravenous Department has inaugurated the system of making rounds.

COLLECTION OF BLOOD SAMPLES

The program for collection of blood samples may be initiated and become an added function of the intravenous department only after

1. The therapists have been adequately trained in the necessary laboratory procedures.
2. A system has been set up for receiving calls.
3. A method has been arranged for transportation of specimens to the laboratories.
4. The nursing staff and the departments have been made aware of their responsibilities.

TRAINING OF THERAPIST. Before this program is initiated, the intravenous therapist should visit the various laboratories. The nurse should be educated in the proper method of collecting, handling, and transporting blood specimens. She must understand and be educated in the performance of the various laboratory tests.

REQUISITIONS. A system for notifying the Intravenous Department of requests for blood samples must be arranged. (1) Requisitions may be sent directly to the Intravenous Department. (2) Requisitions left at a designated area on each floor may be picked up by the intravenous therapist on rounds. This system saves time and prevents the unnecessary handling and sorting of requisitions from all floors.

TRANSPORTATION. A safe method of transporting the specimens to the various laboratories must be arranged. This duty may be allotted to (1) Ward helpers on each floor. (2) Intravenous nurse. This is impractical as many bloods must be delivered to laboratories within a limited time. The accuracy of some tests depends on immediate analysis or proper refrigeration. (3) Messenger service by routine pick up or by call system. (4) By a direct specimen chute to the laboratories.

OPERATIONAL ACTIVITIES OF THE INTRAVENOUS DEPARTMENT AT THE MASSACHUSETTS GENERAL HOSPITAL

Call system

The Intravenous Department has inaugurated the system of routine rounds and makes use of the pagemaster for urgent requests. The department services the wards by means of routine rounds twice a day plus early rounds for fasting blood samples only.

Requests for procedures to be performed are listed with the patient's name and room number on designated blackboards and clipboards. Orders executed are checked off by the therapist. Any orders written after first rounds are added to the board to be carried out on afternoon rounds.

One intravenous nurse in each building is equipped with a pagemaster. This page system is used only when (1) emergency procedures are necessary, (2) urgent procedures are required that must be performed before second rounds, or

(3) tests involving specific times must be made, e.g., blood samples to be drawn at a specific time after injection of dye. The page system is used full time after last rounds are made.

A printed card reading INTRAVENOUS NURSE ON THE FLOOR is carried by each intravenous therapist. This card is left at the desk for the duration of time the nurse is on the ward.

Functions and Regulations of the Intravenous Department

ADMINISTRATION OF PARENTERAL FLUIDS. The intravenous nurse initiates all intravenous infusions, with the exception of those prepared by the doctor and containing drugs not on the authorized list. The intravenous nurse does not

1. Administer intravenous infusions in the lower extremities.
2. Apply positive pressure in administering parenteral fluids.
3. Apply force in administering intravenous or other procedures on rational adult patients. Refusal to comply with treatment is reported to the physician.

The intravenous nurse and the nursing service remove catheter needles and intracatheters when infiltration occurs or infusion is terminated, on the order of the doctor.

PREPARATION AND ADMINISTRATION OF DRUGS IN SOLUTION. The intravenous nurse prepares and administers all drugs on the authorized list only, affixing to the solution bottle a label containing the name of the patient, the name of the drug, dosage prepared, and the time and date. The intravenous nurse must realize that she is legally responsible for every medication she administers.

ADMINISTRATION OF TRANSFUSIONS. The intravenous department initiates transfusions.

1. All transfusions require filters.
2. Bloods are not delivered to the wards until requested by the intravenous therapist.
3. Bloods are not to be placed in the ward refrigerator.
4. Bloods not used within a half hour are to be returned to the blood bank.
5. The intravenous therapist remains and observes the patient for the first 5 minutes after initiating the transfusion.
6. Transfusions are to be terminated at once if reactions occur. *Imperative:* Reaction slips are sent to blood bank with a blood sample.
7. Positive pressure is never applied when administering blood except under the direct supervision of the physician.
8. Staff nurses are not allowed to attach blood to an intravenous infusion. This is the responsibility of the intravenous nurse.

COLLECTION OF VENOUS BLOOD SAMPLES FOR ALL HOSPITAL LABORATORIES. *Program.* Each ward has an allotted area designated for the use of the blood collection program. This area contains:

1. Large envelope in which blood requisitions are left for the intravenous nurse
2. Blood collection equipment, including stock of various Vacutainer tubes and needles
3. Containers (small wire baskets) to hold blood samples, painted different colors to designate the various laboratories

Venous blood samples. All requisitions for venous blood are placed in the requisition envelope until 3 P.M. weekdays and until noon on Saturdays. After 3 P.M. on weekdays only emergency requisitions and requisitions for the blood bank are honored. Each afternoon the intravenous nurse draws blood samples on all surgical admissions, to be sent to the blood bank for typing.

LEVIN TUBES. The intravenous nurse inserts Levin tubes, except that she does not perform this function on patients (1) with esophageal varices, (2) on aneurysm precautions, or (3) who have had radical neck surgery. She does insert Levin tubes for (1) preoperative cases, (2) feeding, (3) gastric analysis, and (4) acid-fast tests.

ADDITIONAL FUNCTIONS. The intravenous therapist also performs *administration of hypodermoclysis, blood volume computation by means of the Volemetron, phlebotomy* (under the supervision of the physician), and (under the direction of the Anesthesia Department) *insertion of intracatheters and central venous pressure catheters* on patients in the operating rooms.

Index